DATE DUE *NH3*

DATE DUE

THE
TOP 1OO RECIPES
for a healthy
LUNCHBOX

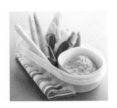

MAR   2008

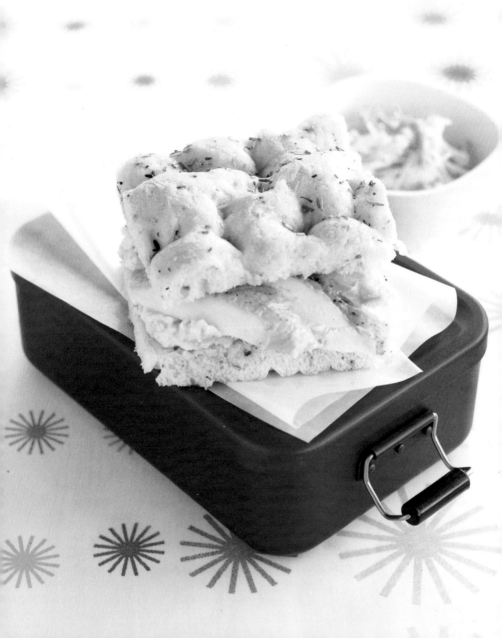

THE
TOP 100 RECIPES
for a healthy
LUNCHBOX

Nicola Graimes

EASY AND EXCITING IDEAS FOR YOUR CHILD'S LUNCHES

DUNCAN BAIRD PUBLISHERS
LONDON

The Top 100 Recipes for a Healthy Lunchbox
Nicola Graimes

Distributed in the USA and Canada by
Sterling Publishing Co., Inc.
387 Park Avenue South, New York, NY 10016-8810

This edition first published in the UK and USA in 2007 by
Duncan Baird Publishers Ltd
Sixth Floor, Castle House
75–76 Wells Street, London W1T 3QH

Managing Editor: Grace Cheetham
Editor: Alison Bolus
Managing Designer: Daniel Sturges
Commissioned photography: David Munn
Food stylist: Bridget Sargeson
Prop stylist: Wei Tang

Library of Congress Cataloging-in-Publication Data Available

ISBN-13: 978-1-84483-507-2   ISBN-10: 1-84483-507-3

10 9 8 7 6 5 4 3 2 1

Typeset in Helvetica Condensed
Color reproduction by Colourscan, Singapore
Printed in China by Imago

To Ella and Joel
I would like to thank Grace Cheetham for
commissioning me to write this book. My
appreciation also goes to Alison Bolus for her
meticulous editing, and the team at DBP.

For information about custom editions, special sales, premium
and corporate purchases, please contact Sterling Special Sales
Department at 800-805-5489 or specialsales@sterlingpub.com.

Publisher's Note
The information in this book is not intended as a substitute for
professional medical advice and treatment. If you are pregnant
or breastfeeding or have any special dietary requirements or
medical conditions, it is recommended that you consult a
medical professional before following any of the information
or recipes contained in this book. Duncan Baird Publishers,
or any other persons who have been involved in working on
this publication, cannot accept responsibility for any errors
or omissions, inadvertent or not, that may be found in the
recipes or text, or for any problems that may arise as a result
of preparing one of these recipes or following the advice
contained in this work.

Notes on the Recipes
Unless otherwise stated:
Use large eggs
Use fresh herbs
1 tsp = 5ml   1 tbsp = 15ml   1 cup = 240ml

Symbols are used to identify even small amounts of an
ingredient, such as the seeds symbol for sunflower oil. Dairy
foods in this book may include cow's, goat's or sheep's milk.
The vegetarian symbol is given to cheeses made using
vegetarian rennet. Please check the manufacturer's labeling
before purchase since some brands may vary. Ensure that
foods are kept chilled until the time of eating, where possible,
and that only the relevantly identified foods are given to those
children with a food allergy or intolerance.

contents

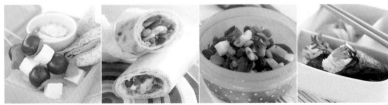

KEY TO SYMBOLS

Suitable for vegetarians: These recipes contain no animal produce, and so can be a good choice for children suffering from inflammatory conditions, such as eczema, asthma and acne, and digestive problems.

Gluten-free: Gluten is the substance in wheat, rye, barley, and oats that adds "stickiness" to baked goods. Gluten intolerance may cause inflammation, depression, and digestive problems. Gluten-free grains include buckwheat and maize.

Wheat-free: Wheat can be difficult to digest. Replace it with maize, buckwheat, rice, tapioca, and rye flours. You can buy wheat-free breads, wraps, and pizza bases.

Dairy-free: Milk can be the cause of nasal blockages and sinusitis, catarrh, and throat and chest infections. It may also trigger conditions such as asthma, eczema, and acne. Try rice, almond, oat, or soy milk.

Contains eggs: If your child has an egg intolerance, it is even more important to give them fresh foods, because egg is often used commercially as a binding agent and thickener. Substitutes for baking are made from arrowroot and agar agar.

Contains nuts: If your child has a nut allergy, you can replace nuts with seeds that you know your child can eat. Never give whole nuts to children under 5, because they can cause choking.

Contains seeds: Pumpkin, sesame, sunflower, and hemp seeds are highly nutritious, but some seeds, particularly sesame, can cause an allergic reaction and so your child may need to avoid them.

INTRODUCTION

For one reason or another, packed lunches seem to throw many of us into a state of panic. The combination of lack of time, early mornings, and a desire to produce a lunch that is varied, interesting, and nutritious and that's not going to come back untouched can be just too much to contemplate five days a week. It's all too easy to slip into a rut when filling a lunchbox, but with a little forward planning and the help of the 100 recipes in this book, you should be inspired.

Lunch is an important meal for everyone but particularly for children, who have high energy requirements for their size. This means that they need nutrient-dense foods in small, regular amounts to keep their bodies and minds working at their best. New evidence suggests a correlation between a child's diet and academic performance. Poor diet is likely to lead to a child with concentration problems, memory difficulties, irritability, and an increased susceptibility to colds and illnesses. By contrast, children who eat regular, healthy meals tend to have more energy, improved learning, and a lower obesity rate.

Tempting as they are, try not to rely on the plethora of prepacked, processed foods specifically aimed at children's lunchboxes. Most are not only wasteful due to excessive packaging but also contain high amounts of salt, saturated or hydrogenated fat, sugar, additives, and preservatives; it will come as no surprise that these foods have a negative effect, not only on our children's health but on the environment too. It's all too easy to get sucked in by their overwhelming colorful presence in supermarkets. Recent research in the U.K. found that only one in five lunchboxes is healthy enough to meet government standards, and the U.K. is not alone in this situation.

ABOUT THIS BOOK

The main aim of this book is to inspire: The majority of the recipes are quick and easy to prepare; others take a little more forethought and preparation but can be made in bulk and frozen for future use. Many of the recipes will also keep for a few days in the refrigerator, allowing you to plan ahead and ease the morning pressure.

The emphasis is on good-quality, wholesome fresh food without being puritanical—you will find, therefore, some recipes for sweet treats. Many of these contain fruit; try to avoid giving those that

don't to your child every day, although it's not necessary to avoid them altogether —there's nothing more tempting than a food that's not allowed! The same goes for potato chips—give them as an occasional treat and choose brands that are made with good, honest ingredients, avoid overly colored snacks, and steer clear of those that contain a long list of additives. You will notice that the recipes in this book are not full of suggestions to switch to low-fat this or "lite" that. Why? Because many of these foods may indeed be lower in fat than the original article, but they invariably contain additives to compensate for the lack of taste. A food is not necessarily healthy just because it's low in fat and, strangely, some low-fat foods contain bucketloads of sugar. Obviously our children's diets should not be overloaded with saturated or hydrogenated fat, sugar, and salt, but it's equally important to eat foods that have been produced with care and consideration, such as free-range, organic, and Fairtrade foods.

Each recipe comes with an explanation of its health benefits as well as some serving suggestions, enabling you to create a nutritionally balanced and varied lunchbox on a daily basis. Use the serving suggestions as a guide: You don't have to stick to them religiously, because obviously likes and dislikes as well as the foods you have to hand will influence what you decide to pack in the lunchbox. As for portion sizes, these are averages only, since the size of meals you need to make will obviously differ widely depending on whether you have a picky 5 year old or a ravenous teenager.

The recipes have been created to appeal to both adults and children. While being devised as part of a packed lunch for a child, they could equally be taken to the office, form part of a picnic, or be eaten at home for lunch; many of the recipes would also make a welcome after school supper.

SPECIAL DIETS

If your child is a vegetarian or vegan, has an allergy to nuts, or an intolerance of dairy products, eggs, wheat, or gluten, you will need to take more care when preparing their lunchboxes. The symbols shown on page 6 are used throughout the book to indicate which recipes are safe for particular diets, and the menu plans provided on pages 140–143 give ideas for a week's worth of lunchboxes for some of these diets.

PLANNING AHEAD

Planning ahead makes preparing a lunchbox so much easier. Not only does it relieve the daily panic of what to include, but it also makes the weekly shop more straightforward. This is the perfect time to get your child involved too by giving them the opportunity to choose foods that they would like in their lunchbox, on the premise that they are more likely to eat what they have selected or helped to prepare.

Write down a daily menu for the week ahead, referring to pages 140–143 for guidelines or to use as a template. The menu can be made up of fresh fruit and vegetables, freshly prepared foods, some preprepared and frozen dishes, as well as those invaluable leftovers.

When you are deciding on what to cook for dinner, think how you can incorporate leftovers into a lunch the following day, or just cook a bit extra. The following foods have potential as leftovers and make excellent additions to a lunchbox:

- Pasta, rice, potatoes, couscous, bulgur wheat, or pearl barley (but note that you should keep cooked rice and grains no longer than two days in the refrigerator to avoid any danger of food poisoning)
- Meat and poultry—chicken, turkey, beef, lamb, or pork, or any type of sausage
- Fish and shellfish—broiled/griddled tuna, salmon or trout, shrimp or squid
- Vegetables—roasted or broiled

- Eggs—soft or hard-boiled, omelet, frittata, or tortilla
- Undressed salads
- Soup
- Fruit—sauces, compotes, salads

CHOOSING A LUNCHBOX

There is plenty of choice when looking for a lunchbox, and your child will probably want to be involved in choosing their favorite, whether it be an attractive color or decorated with a popular cartoon character. It's an important consideration to make, since a lunchbox can often make or break the success of a packed lunch—an embarrassing, age-inappropriate design is simply not "cool" enough to be seen with!

- Make sure the lunchbox is sturdy, the handle is strong enough to withstand being swung around, and the box can be opened and closed easily by a child.
- Insure the lunchbox is insulated and/or comes with an ice pack if your child

does not have access to a refrigerator at school. This is important for cooked meat, eggs, dairy foods, seafood, rice, couscous, and bulgur wheat salads, which should all ideally be kept cold until lunchtime. Many lunchboxes come with a separate pocket or section in which the ice pack can be inserted so that it doesn't touch the contents.

- Make sure the lunchbox is large enough to hold a drink bottle, or Thermos for the winter. Warm the Thermos first by filling it with just-boiled water 15 minutes.

- Think about waste, too: You can now buy lunchboxes that come with lidded containers that fit snuggly within the external case, which can be reused rather than thrown away every day, eliminating the need for excessive packaging, including plastic wrap and foil.

- Make sure the lunchbox is easy to clean and that there are no nooks and crannies that are tricky to get at.

PRESENTATION

A little attention to detail can make a big difference to a lunchbox's appeal. Plastic tubs come in a range of shapes, sizes, and colors and are perfect for dips, crudités, kebabs, salads, fruit, sandwiches, and wraps. Avoid foods that are likely to break up or be damaged during transit (remember the mushy black banana that returns untouched!). Just including a range of different colored foods, especially fruit and vegetables, will add to its appeal.

BALANCING ACT

It may come as little surprise to learn that according to recent research the most popular items in a lunchbox are a sliced white bread sandwich with a filling of ham, cheese, or chicken; potato chips; a chocolate bar or cookie; and a yogurt or cheese snack. While, there's nothing intrinsically wrong with any of these foods on an occasional basis, if a child eats them every day, they will not get the range of nutrients they need for good health. The key to a healthy packed lunch is nutritional balance and a wide variety of foods.

To make things easier, use the following guidelines as a template for your child's lunchbox. They show the importance of offering a variety of foods from the main food groups. By following these suggestions you can insure your lunchbox provides the foods your child needs for health, development, and well-being.

PUTTING IT INTO PRACTICE

A nutritionally balanced lunchbox should feature one or more items from each of the following food groups.

Fruit and vegetables

- Many of us struggle to get our kids to eat enough fruit and vegetables a day, yet the lunchbox provides the perfect opportunity to boost a child's consumption of fresh produce. Choose different types, which not only insures your child gets a range of nutrients but also helps to avoid the boredom factor.

- Consider presenting fruit in different ways: in a fruit salad, compote, pureed, chopped, sliced, and so on. Look out for mini-packs of dried fruit, but do check the label first because some contain additives as well as added sugar and fat. Better still, make your own mixes, incorporating shredded coconut, nuts, and seeds, which add vital nutrients.

- Children often prefer raw vegetables to cooked: cherry tomatoes or sticks of carrot, cucumber and bell pepper are popular, but you could also try slices of fennel, flowerets of broccoli and cauliflower, fresh peas, whole snow peas, sugar snap peas, baby corn, and salad leaves. Certain vegetables are best cooked, such as asparagus, beets, and green beans.

Dairy foods

- About half of adult bone density is laid down during adolescence, so it is important to provide good sources of calcium, such as dairy foods. Many of the cheeses for lunchboxes are of the processed variety—dippers, dunkers, strings, etc. Do check labels first but, better still, a healthier and cheaper option is to include a chunk of farmhouse cheese, preferably organic. Bear in mind that many cheeses are high in saturated fat so use in moderation or opt for lower-fat alternatives such as low-fat cream cheese, mozzarella, feta, and Brie. (Nondairy sources of calcium include green leafy vegetables, sardines, eggs, nuts, seeds, and wholegrain cereals.)

- Look at the label on a fruit yogurt and you may find that it contains very little real fruit, if any, and then you have the additional undesirable sweeteners, sugar, colors, and preservatives. To make your own fruit yogurt, simply puree or finely chop some fresh fruit and blend it with a cupful of thick and creamy natural bio yogurt, and a teaspoonful of clear honey or maple syrup if the fruit is a little tart. Yogurt, like fromage frais, is a first-class protein food, while bio versions contain "good" bacteria that benefit the digestive system. Adding a tablespoonful of toasted oats and seeds further boosts the vitamin and mineral content.

Protein

- Protein foods are great for staving off hunger pangs and work in unison with carbohydrate foods, which provide long term energy and help to boost concentration, memory, and attention span. Use protein rich foods in sandwich fillings, savory dishes, and salads or to nibble on. Good examples are: lean, cooked chicken, turkey, or beef; fish and shrimp; eggs; nuts, nut butters, and seeds; legumes and hummus; vegetarian sausages and nut cutlets; tofu.

- Children in particular need omega-3 essential fatty acids for their developing brains, eyes, and nerves. Omega-3 has also been shown to improve mood and benefit those with dyslexia and attention deficit hyperactivity disorder. Types of oily fish include herring, salmon, trout, mackerel, sardines, and tuna, which all make great sandwich fillings, pâtés, savory dishes, and salads.

Starchy carbs

- Whole grains are the body's main source of long-term energy and should be at the heart of a lunchbox. Bread is the obvious option and there are now so many different types to choose from: ditch white bread in favor of brown or rye for healthy sandwiches; fill rolls, buns, and bagels; use pita breads as pockets or cut into strips for dipping; and use flat breads to wrap around fillings. Cookie cutters are a great way to make different shaped sandwiches, adding extra interest for young eaters.

- Alternatively, try rice, noodles, or potatoes. They all make a great base for a salad and hold up well to being transported. Combine cooked pasta or rice with diced red bell pepper, canned corn, fresh tomato, and cubes of cheese, and lubricate with a spoonful of pesto and reduced-fat mayonnaise. Couscous and bulgur wheat are great with chopped tomato, cucumber, scallion, olives, and mint, then dressed with lemon juice and olive oil. Cooked noodles work with oriental-style dressings, such as a mix of soy sauce, sesame oil, and fresh ginger.

Drinks

Most children don't drink enough fluids, especially while at school. Dehydration can affect concentration and intellectual performance, as well as the transportation of nutrients around the body. A 2 percent loss in body fluids, for example, can cause a 20 percent reduction in both physical and mental performance. Make sure you provide a bottle of water, diluted fresh fruit juice, or milk, and avoid carbonated and other sugary drinks. Most fruit drinks contain little in the way of fruit and lots of sugar, so opt for freshly squeezed instead and dilute with a little water.

If you find it difficult to get your child to drink water, fresh fruit smoothies and vegetable juices are a nutritious alternative and count as one portion out of the recommended servings of fruit and vegetables a day. There are plenty to choose from in the chiller cabinets of most supermarkets or they are simple to make at home: Blend a banana with natural yogurt and a little milk for an energy sustaining drink. Strawberries, nectarines, raspberries, and mango are also good alternatives for a summery flavor. For a vegetable version, apple, carrot, and beet is a colorful and tasty combination.

SHOPPING LIST

Ideally, lunchboxes should be appealing, inviting, "cool" enough to withstand scrutiny from peers, and never boring! If this sounds a tall order, then forward planning and organization make it that much easier. The first step is shopping —keep a list in the kitchen of what you need to buy for the week. Break the list down into various food types, including fresh foods with a limited shelf life, breads, chilled foods, frozen foods, and pantry staples. Arming yourself with a list when shopping will also give you the strength to stand firm against pester power: "If it's not on the list, I'm not going to buy it!"

The following lists of foods make a helpful guide and a good starting point.

Fresh fruit and vegetables

These have a limited shelf life, so try to avoid wastage by not buying too much. Buy as fresh as possible and, if you can, opt for organic, seasonal fruit and vegetables. Make the most of local markets, farmer's markets, and delivery boxes.

Choose from fruits such as kiwi fruit, melons, mangoes, pineapples, apples, grapes, citrus fruits, bananas, pears, nectarines, peaches, plums, strawberries, raspberries, and blueberries. Also offer your child avocados, salad leaves, bell peppers, carrots, corn, broccoli, cauliflower, scallions, tomatoes, beet, celery, cucumber, soybeans, green beans, potatoes, sweet potatoes, herbs, squash, and sprouted seeds and beans.

Chilled foods

The following foods have a limited shelf life, so buy regularly in small amounts. These protein foods make a valuable contribution to a lunchbox, keeping hunger pangs at bay for the afternoon ahead. However, some are high in fat, so it's best to keep an eye on food labels and opt for lower fat varieties. Nutritional chilled foods to choose from are: eggs, tofu, hummus, guacamole, dips, pâtés and spreads, deli meat such as ham, salami, cooked chicken, and so on, sausages, fish and shellfish, cheese, soup, mayonnaise, olives/sun-dried tomatoes, natural bio yogurt, fromage frais, rice pudding, fruit juice, and smoothies.

Pantry

Most of these foods will keep for weeks or months and can readily form a central part of a lunchbox, so it's a good idea to keep a good selection. Keep an eye on best before and use-by dates and note that some products require chilling after opening.

The range is very wide, but here are some of the many foods that will form the backbone of your lunchbox ingredients:

KEEP IT SAFE

When preparing a lunchbox, pay special care to food safety and hygiene. Keep all foods, and especially those susceptible to food poisoning bacteria, such as meat, poultry, fish, dairy, eggs, rice, and other grains, well chilled. Pack in an insulated lunchbox with an ice pack or store in the refrigerator, if possible.

Breads

Bread is most nutritious when made with wholewheat flour and also contains a higher amount of fiber. Try different varieties of bread to avoid the boredom factor and store a supply of bread in the freezer to avoid running out: wholewheat bread, bagels, pita breads, focaccias, ciabattas, rolls, flatbreads, baguettes, fruit bread, muffins, scones, and currant buns.

Frozen

Frozen food can be a valuable asset when preparing a lunchbox. Freeze homemade soups and other prepared foods in single portions for future use. Frozen fruits and vegetables make a convenient standby and are often more nutritious than fresh, having been frozen soon after picking. Purees, compotes, and sauces all freeze well. Choose vegetables, fruit, fish/shellfish, meat, soup, tarts, pies, bread, pizza, homemade burgers, falafel, and potato cakes.

dried fruit (try to avoid those with added sugar and sulfur dioxide, because this can exacerbate asthma), canned fruit, rice cakes, crackers, breadsticks, corn crackers, tortillas, couscous, bulgur wheat, barley, pasta, noodles, polenta, rice, canned beans and lentils, canned fish, nuts and seeds, flour, canned tomatoes and corn, pesto, herbs and spices, oats, nut butters, honey, high-fruit/low-sugar jam, pretzels, popcorn, and low-sugar cereal bars.

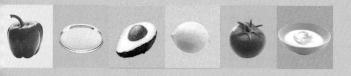

NIBBLES & DIPS

The varied recipes within this chapter will all add substance and variety with the minimum of effort or time—all positive attributes when making a lunchbox. They are also a way to get extra nutrition into children. Many children love to eat with their fingers, and a selection of vegetable sticks are perfect for dunking into healthy dips such as hummus, guacamole, and tzatziki. While the Smoked Salmon Pâté and Smashed Bean & Carrot Spread can be dipped into too, they are also delicious spread over pita bread or crispbread. Presentation is a key factor in the success of a lunchbox, and "things on sticks," such as Mozzarella, Cherry Tomato & Basil, or Salami, Cheese & Pineapple, will tempt even the fussiest of eaters.

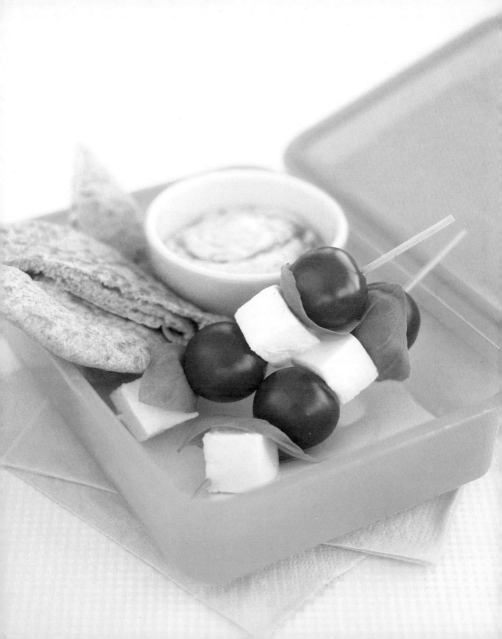

soy-coated nuts & seeds

Store-bought roasted nuts are generally deep-fried. Here the nuts and seeds are roasted without any fat, then lightly sprinkled with soy sauce. If nuts are a no-no, increase the seeds.

SERVES 4

PREPARATION + COOKING
5 + 10 minutes

STORAGE
Make in advance and keep in an airtight container for up to 1 week.

SERVE THIS WITH...
Pear & Ham Bundles
(see page 24)
Tabbouleh (see page 90)
fruit yogurt
fruit

HEALTH BENEFITS
Yes, nuts are high in fat but, on the whole, it is the healthy monounsaturated type. They're also rich in protein, calcium, iron, vitamin E, selenium, and fiber. Seeds are good too, with pumpkin providing both omega-3 and omega-6 fats.

scant 2 cups mixed unsalted nuts and seeds: peanuts (skins rubbed off), almonds, cashews, walnuts, hazelnuts, brazils, sunflower, hemp, pumpkin, or linseeds
1–2 tsp. soy sauce

1 Heat the oven to 325°F. Place the nuts on a baking sheet and roast about 6 minutes. Add the seeds and roast another 2–4 minutes until they smell toasted and are golden; watch carefully because they burn easily.
2 Remove from the oven and transfer to a bowl. Let cool slightly then drizzle with the soy sauce, turning the nuts and seeds with a spoon until they are coated.

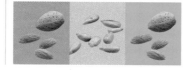

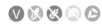

savory spicy popcorn

Delicious as it is, popcorn doesn't have to be smothered in caramel or salt. For a healthier version, it's easy to make your own low-fat, sugar-free, salt-free alternative.

1 tbsp. sunflower oil
2½oz. popping corn

1 tsp. Cajun spice mix

1 Heat the oil in a saucepan, then add the popping corn in a single layer. Cover the pan with a lid and cook over medium heat, shaking the pan frequently, until the corn has popped. Do not lift the lid until it has finished popping.
2 Transfer the popcorn to a large bowl and sprinkle the spice mix over the top. Turn the popcorn with a spoon until it is coated in the spices. Let cool.

SERVES 4

PREPARATION + COOKING
2 + 3 minutes

STORAGE
Make in advance and keep in an airtight container for up to 3 days.

SERVE THIS WITH...
Cool Dogs (see page 69)
salad
Strawberry Crunch Cup
 (see page 124)
fruit

HEALTH BENEFITS
Corn is one of the most nutritionally balanced carbohydrate foods and provides plenty of long-term energy.

cheesy celery stalks

A stalk of celery makes a natural container for cream cheese or any type of pâté or thick dip. A halved and cored apple, pear, or seeded cucumber would also work well.

SERVES 1

PREPARATION
5 minutes

STORAGE
Make on the day.

SERVE THIS WITH...
Roast Chicken & Avocado
  Focaccia (see page 67)
Winter Fruit Salad
  (see page 122), pureed
fruit yogurt

HEALTH BENEFITS
Celery was grown as a medicinal plant before it was even considered a food. Traditionally, it was used to treat nervousness, but it can also help to curb high blood pressure.

1 stalk celery
1–2 tbsp. low-fat cream cheese
    (flavor of choice)

1 Cut the celery in half or thirds, depending on its length.
2 Spread the cream cheese into the groove running down the stalks of celery.

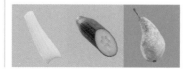

honey-sesame sausages

Buy the best quality sausages you can, with a high meat content, preferably organic. Small cocktail sausages are easy for children to eat: serve in a tub or on some lettuce or cucumber.

2 tsp. olive oil
1 tbsp. honey
1 tsp. Dijon mustard

12 good quality
   cocktail sausages
1 tsp. sesame seeds (optional)

1 Heat the oven to 350°F. Mix together the oil, honey, and mustard in a bowl. Add the sausages and turn to coat them in the mixture.
2 Arrange the sausages in a nonstick roasting pan and cook in the oven about 12–14 minutes, turning occasionally, until almost cooked. Sprinkle the sesame seeds over, if using, and cook another minute until the sausages are golden and cooked through. Let cool.

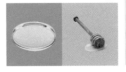

SERVES 2–4

PREPARATION + COOKING
5 + 15 minutes

STORAGE
Make in advance and refrigerate for up to 3 days. Keep chilled until ready to eat (see page 11).

SERVE THIS WITH...
Tzatziki (see page 34)
Cheese, Apple & Chutney Bun (see page 52)
natural yogurt with honey
fruit

HEALTH BENEFITS
Red meat is classed as a first-class protein, meaning that it provides all the amino acids required by the body for its growth and repair. It's also a good source of iron, and studies have found that children are often deficient in this mineral, which can influence behavior and development.

pear & ham bundles

SERVES 1

PREPARATION
5 minutes

STORAGE
Make on the day. Keep chilled until ready to eat (see page 11).

SERVE THIS WITH…
Italian Flag Salad (see page 80)
chunk of bread
Apricot Cookie (see page 136)
fruit

HEALTH BENEFITS
Pears are one of the least allergenic of foods and are therefore excellent for children. Full of natural sweetness, pears also provide vitamin C, and fiber if the skin is left on.

Pear is a natural partner to Parma ham, as is melon, nectarine, or peach. These bundles make a change from the obvious sandwich, and you could carry on the Italian theme with an Italian Flag Salad (see page 80) and a chunk of ciabatta. Alternatively, you could try wrapping the ham around some breadsticks.

1 ripe but not too soft pear,
   quartered and cored

squeeze of lemon juice
2 slices Parma ham, halved

1 Place the pear quarters on a plate, squeeze the lemon juice over them, and turn until they are coated—this will help to prevent them browning.
2 Wrap one strip of Parma ham around each pear quarter.

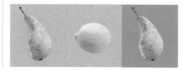

mozzarella, cherry tomato & basil sticks

Attractive presentation can perk up a tired looking lunchbox, and these colorful kebabs take only minutes to make. For young children, omit the sticks and serve in a small tub.

4 cherry tomatoes
4 basil leaves
4 (½in.) cubes
   mozzarella cheese

Pesto dip:
2 tbsp. low-fat natural
   bio yogurt
2 tsp. green pesto

1 To make the dip, mix together the yogurt and pesto then spoon into a small lidded container.
2 Thread a cherry tomato onto a toothpick, followed by a basil leaf and a cube of mozzarella. Repeat with a second tomato, basil leaf, and cube of mozzarella, then assemble a second stick. Serve the toothpicks with the pesto dip.

SERVES 1

PREPARATION
10 minutes

STORAGE
Make the dip in advance and refrigerate for up to 1 week. Assemble the sticks on the day.

SERVE THIS WITH...
slices of wholewheat pita bread
carrot sticks
Date & Pecan Brownie
  (see page 133)
fruit

HEALTH BENEFITS
Mozzarella is relatively low in fat but still provides valuable amounts of bone-building calcium—vital for growing kids.

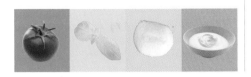

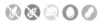

chicken strips with satay dip

Full of appetite satisfying protein, these chicken sticks and peanut dip are fun to eat and easy to make. Tzatziki (page 34) or Tomato Salsa (page 30) can be served instead of the satay dip if peanuts are not allowed in your child's school.

SERVES 1

PREPARATION + COOKING
10 + 6 minutes

STORAGE
Make in advance and refrigerate the dip for up to 1 week and the chicken for up to 3 days. Keep chilled until ready to eat (see page 11).

SERVE THIS WITH...
carrot, cucumber, and
 bell pepper sticks
wholewheat tortilla
Apricot Cookie (see page 136)
fruit

HEALTH BENEFITS
Chicken is an excellent source of low-fat protein and is a good source of selenium, which helps to support the immune system.

1 tbsp. olive oil
1 tsp. paprika
5oz. skinless chicken breast,
 cut into 4–6 strips

Satay dip:
2 tbsp. peanut butter

1 tsp. olive oil
1 tsp. tamari (wheat free
 soy sauce)
½ tsp. soft light brown sugar
1 tbsp. reduced-fat coconut
 milk or mayonnaise

1 To make the satay dip, mix together all the ingredients with 1 tablespoon of hot water in a bowl until combined, then transfer to a lidded cup.

2 Put the oil in a shallow dish, add the paprika and then the chicken. Turn the chicken in the oil.

3 Heat a large skillet and fry the chicken about 2–3 minutes on each side until golden and cooked through. Let cool.

4 Serve the strips dipped into the satay sauce.

salami, cheese & pineapple sticks

A twist on the favorite cheese and pineapple combination. If you have fresh pineapple, so much the better, because it tends to be richer in vitamins than the canned version, although this is more than adequate, especially if it is canned in natural juice.

4 thin slices salami
4 chunks pineapple

4 large bite-size cubes cheddar or other hard cheese

1 Fold a slice of salami in half, then half again, and thread onto a toothpick, followed by a chunk of pineapple, then a chunk of cheddar.
2 Repeat to make four sticks.

MAKES 4

PREPARATION
5 minutes

STORAGE
Make the day before and refrigerate. Keep chilled until ready to eat (see page 11).

SERVE THIS WITH...
Mixed Bean Salad (see page 82)
Custard Tartlet (see page 135)
fruit

HEALTH BENEFITS
Pineapple aids digestion, particularly that of protein foods, and has also been found to have antiinflammatory properties.

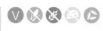

*roasted red bell pepper hummus

HEALTH BENEFITS
Chickpeas are low in fat and a good source of both protein and carbohydrate. As an added bonus, they count as one of the recommended portions of fruit and vegetables we should eat each day.

Hummus is a versatile addition to a lunchbox. It makes a perfect dip with vegetable sticks or a sandwich filling. In addition, a spoonful can be added to soups. The roasted red bell pepper adds flavor and color.

1 red bell pepper, seeded
  and quartered
3 tbsp. extra-virgin olive oil,
  plus extra for drizzling
1½ cups canned no-salt,
  no-sugar chickpeas, drained
  and rinsed

2 cloves garlic, halved
1 heaped tbsp. light tahini
  (sesame seed paste)
juice of ½ lemon
salt
freshly ground black pepper

SERVES 6

PREPARATION + COOKING
15 + 30 minutes

STORAGE
Make in advance and refrigerate
for up to 1 week.

SERVE THIS WITH...
vegetable sticks, such as red
  bell pepper, cucumber, carrot,
  sugar snap peas, and baby corn
seeded breadsticks
Ham & Egg Pie (see page 103)
fruit yogurt
fruit

1 Heat the oven to 400°F. Put the bell pepper quarters in a roasting pan with 1 tablespoon of the oil. Toss the bell pepper in the oil until coated, then roast 25–30 minutes, turning once, until the skin begins to blister and blacken.
2 Remove the bell pepper from the oven and leave until cool enough to handle, then peel off the skin.
3 Put the bell pepper in a food processor or blender with the chickpeas, garlic, tahini, lemon juice, 2 tablespoons of water, and the rest of the oil. Blend until the mixture forms a chunky, creamy puree, occasionally scraping the mixture down the sides of the processor or blender.
4 Transfer the hummus to a lidded container. Season to taste and drizzle a little extra olive oil over the top.

> **Garlic is known for its heart protecting properties and is most potent when raw.**

tortilla dippers with tomato salsa

Crispy tortillas are delicious dunked into this rich salsa or some Roasted Red Bell Pepper Hummus (see page 28), Creamy Guacamole (see page 31), or Tzatziki (see page 34).

1 wholewheat tortilla
1 tsp. olive oil

Tomato salsa:
2 tbsp. olive oil
2 cloves garlic, crushed

1½ cups passata (strained tomatoes)
1 tbsp. sun-dried tomato paste
½ tsp. sugar
2 tomatoes, seeded and cut into small pieces (optional)

1 To make the tomato salsa, heat the oil in a saucepan. Fry the garlic 1 minute, stirring to prevent it burning. Add the passata, tomato paste, and sugar, then bring to a boil. Reduce the heat to low, half-cover the pan with a lid and simmer 15 minutes. Stir the sauce occasionally to prevent it sticking to the bottom of the pan. Let cool then stir in the fresh tomatoes, if using.

2 Cut the tortilla in half and then into three or four wedges depending on its size. Heat the oil in a skillet and fry the wedges in batches about 2 minutes on each side until golden and crisp. When cool, pack with the salsa.

SERVES 1 (SALSA FOR 4)

PREPARATION + COOKING
10 + 20 minutes

STORAGE
Make the salsa in advance and refrigerate for up to 3 days or freeze for up to 1 month. Cook the tortilla wedges on the day.

SERVE THIS WITH...
Honey-sesame Sausages (see page 23)
Apple Coleslaw (see page 76)
muffin
fruit

HEALTH BENEFITS
Tomatoes contain antioxidants, including significant amounts of vitamins E and C and beta-carotene, which have a protective effect on the body. Canned tomatoes have similar nutritional values to fresh.

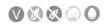

creamy guacamole

Raw vegetables are often more acceptable to children than cooked, and even the most unlikely of veg are good served in this way. Try extending the choice from bell peppers, carrots, and cucumbers to cauliflower, broccoli, snow peas, and baby corn. If time allows, make the guacamole on the day of serving because it is best as fresh as possible.

1 ripe avocado, halved and pit removed
1 clove garlic, crushed
juice of ½ small lemon or juice of 1 lime
1 tbsp. mayonnaise
1 tbsp. finely chopped fresh cilantro (optional)
salt
freshly ground black pepper

1 Use a spoon to scoop the avocado out of its skin into a bowl. Stir in the garlic, lemon or lime juice, and mayonnaise and mash using a fork to achieve the consistency you want.
2 Stir in the cilantro, if using, and season to taste.

SERVES 4

PREPARATION
10 minutes

STORAGE
Make the day before and refrigerate overnight, or make on the day.

SERVE THIS WITH....
vegetable sticks, such as snow peas, baby corn and broccoli flowerets
Falafel & Hummus Lavash (see page 68), replacing the hummus
Carrot Cake (see page 134)
fruit

HEALTH BENEFITS
Avocados have recently been found to be a good source of lutein, which protects the eyes against disease such as cataracts and age-related degeneration.

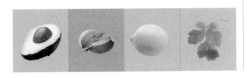

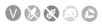

roasted eggplant dip

If your child doesn't usually like eggplant, then why not try it in this slightly spicy, garlicky dip? It's good spread on pita bread or dipped into with breadsticks and vegetable sticks.

SERVES 4–6

PREPARATION + COOKING
15 + 40 minutes

STORAGE
Make in advance and refrigerate for up to 5 days.

SERVE THIS WITH...
breadsticks or pita bread slices
carrot, cucumber, celery, and/or sweet bell pepper sticks
Spicy Sweet Potatoes (see page 95)
fruit

HEALTH BENEFITS
Look for bright, shiny, firm eggplants, which will be a richer source of vitamins B and C than those that are past their best.

1 large eggplant
2 cloves garlic
1 tbsp. light tahini (sesame seed paste)
1 tsp. ground cumin
1 tsp. ground coriander
2 tbsp. extra-virgin olive oil
juice of ½ lemon
salt
freshly ground black pepper

1 Heat the oven to 400°F. Prick the eggplant all over with a fork then place in a roasting pan. Roast about 40 minutes until the inside of the eggplant is very soft.
2 Leave to cool slightly then halve the eggplant lengthwise and scoop out the flesh with a spoon into a food processor or blender. Add the garlic, tahini, spices, olive oil, and lemon juice. Process until smooth and creamy. Season to taste.

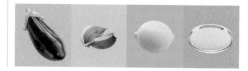

smashed bean & carrot spread

Lima beans have a bit of an image problem, but if combined with stronger flavors such as spices they make a great base for a spread.

1 carrot, sliced
2 tbsp. extra-virgin olive oil
2 cloves garlic, crushed
1 tsp. ground cumin
¼ tsp. ground cinnamon
1 tsp. ground coriander

2 pinches chili powder
1½ cups canned lima
   beans, drained and rinsed
juice of 1 lemon
salt
freshly ground black pepper

1 Steam the carrot until tender. Meanwhile, heat the oil in a saucepan and fry the garlic and spices 1 minute. Add the beans, lemon juice, and 2–3 tablespoons of water, then heat gently, stirring.
2 Put the carrot in a food processor or blender with the bean mixture. Process until smooth, adding a little extra water if necessary, then season to taste.

SERVES 4–6

PREPARATION + COOKING
10 + 5 minutes

STORAGE
Make in advance and refrigerate for up to 5 days.

TRY THIS WITH...
pita bread or flatbread
Melon & Halloumi Salad
  (see page 78)
cookie

HEALTH BENEFITS
Canned beans are not only convenient but also a good source of low-fat protein, fiber, iron, magnesium, and B vitamins.

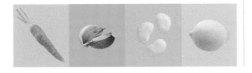

tzatziki

This Greek dip is traditionally made using yogurt and cucumber, flavored with mint, and served with pita bread. This version uses low-fat natural bio yogurt and finely grated zucchini, which contains less water than cucumber and so holds together better.

SERVES 2

PREPARATION
10 minutes

STORAGE
Make in advance and refrigerate for up to 3 days.

SERVE THIS WITH...
wholewheat pita bread
Falafel (see page 104)
Apple Flapjack (see page 126)
fruit

HEALTH BENEFITS
Studies show that certain cultures in yogurt may help to boost immunity, protect against infection, and support the digestive system by increasing the amount of "friendly" bacteria in the gut.

4 tbsp. low-fat natural bio yogurt
2in. piece zucchini, finely grated

1 small clove garlic, crushed
2 tbsp. finely chopped mint
salt
freshly ground black pepper

1 Mix together the yogurt, zucchini, garlic, and mint in a lidded container or bowl.
2 Season to taste.

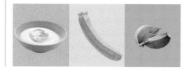

smoked salmon pâté

Children are recommended to eat at least one portion of oily fish a week, and this creamy smoked salmon pâté is ideal and simple to prepare. You could use smoked mackerel or smoked trout as an alternative.

6oz. smoked salmon pieces
juice of ½ lemon, or to taste
¼ lb. low-fat cream cheese

½ tsp. paprika
freshly ground black pepper

1 Put the salmon, lemon juice, cream cheese, and paprika into a blender or food processor. Process until smooth and creamy. Season with pepper to taste.
2 Transfer to a bowl, cover, and put in the refrigerator.

SERVES ABOUT 6

PREPARATION
10 minutes

STORAGE
Make in advance and refrigerate for up to 3 days. Keep chilled until ready to eat (see page 11).

SERVE THIS WITH...
Oat Crackers (see page 137)
cherry tomatoes and
  cucumber sticks
Carrot Cake (see page 134)
fruit

HEALTH BENEFITS
Smoked salmon is a rich source of omega-3 essential fatty acids, which benefit a child's developing brain, eyes and nervous system.

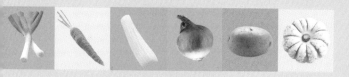

SOUPS

Soup makes a fantastic addition to a lunchbox—wholesome, warming, versatile, and nutritious. The colder winter months can put parents off packed lunches in favor of a warm school meal, but many lunchboxes now come with a small unbreakable flask, allowing soup to be taken to school. Soups keep well and are ideal for making in advance: either chill or freeze in portions and reheat on the day. Chunky homemade vegetable, bean, pasta, or noodle soups make a complete meal, providing protein and carbohydrates. Pureed soups are great for children who dislike "bits" or won't eat vegetables, since the smooth texture disguises the ingredients. To make a nutritious and balanced lunch, just add some bread and a chunk of cheese or slice of cold meat.

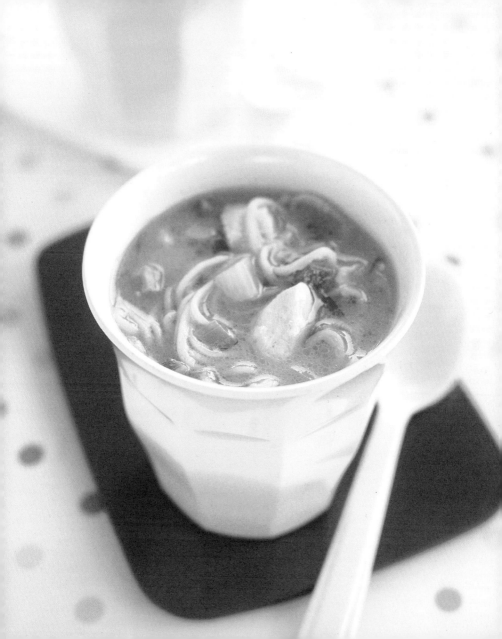

creamy tomato & lentil soup

Tomato is many children's favorite soup. This version contains a nutritional boost, thanks to the lentils, which become hidden when cooked.

SERVES 4

PREPARATION + COOKING
15 + 35 minutes

STORAGE
Make in advance and refrigerate for up to 3 days or freeze in single portions.

SERVE THIS WITH...
onion bagel
Strawberry Crunch Cup
  (see page 124)
dried apricots

HEALTH BENEFITS
Tomatoes get their color from a natural plant compound called lycopene, which is best absorbed by the body when tomatoes are cooked. Lycopene has been found to protect us from some cancers and heart disease.

½ cup split red lentils
1 tbsp. olive oil
1 large onion, chopped
1 carrot, chopped
1²/₃ cups passata (strained tomatoes)

3¾ cups gluten-free vegetable stock
1 bay leaf
4 tbsp. reduced-fat crème fraîche
salt and ground black pepper

1 Rinse the lentils, put in a saucepan, cover with water, and bring to a boil. Reduce the heat and simmer, half-covered, 15 minutes until tender. Drain and set aside.
2 Meanwhile, heat the oil in a large saucepan. Add the onion and fry, half-covered, 7 minutes, then add the carrot. Fry the vegetables, half-covered, another 3 minutes, stirring occasionally.
3 Add the passata, stock, cooked lentils, and bay leaf. Bring to a boil, then reduce the heat and simmer, part-covered, 20 minutes until the vegetables are tender.
4 Puree in a blender or using a hand blender. Stir in the crème fraîche, season, and heat through gently.

green giant soup

Petits pois have a delicate sweet flavor and tender outer skin that work well in this vibrantly colored green soup.

1 tbsp. olive oil
1 large leek, finely chopped
1 stalk celery, thinly sliced
1 bay leaf
2 large sprigs mint (optional)
2 potatoes, peeled and cubed

5 cups gluten-free vegetable stock
heaped 2 cups frozen petits pois
½ cup milk (optional)

1 Heat the oil in a large saucepan and fry the leek 5 minutes until softened. Add the celery, bay leaf, mint, if using, and potatoes and cook, half-covered, 3 minutes.
2 Pour in the stock and bring to a boil. Reduce the heat, half-cover, and simmer 20 minutes. Add the peas and cook another 5 minutes until the vegetables are tender.
3 Puree in a blender or using a hand blender. Return to the pan and stir in the milk, if using, or more stock, and heat through gently. Season to taste.

SERVES 4

PREPARATION + COOKING
10 + 25 minutes

STORAGE
Make in advance and refrigerate for up to 3 days or freeze in single portions.

SERVE THIS WITH...
strips of crispy broiled bacon to dip in or to crush and sprinkle over the top
Cheese Scones (see page 138)
fruit

HEALTH BENEFITS
Little nuggets of goodness, frozen peas are often richer in nutrients than fresh ones.
A good source of protein and fiber, peas also provide iron, vitamins C and B, and folate.

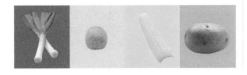

corn chowder

SERVES 4

PREPARATION + COOKING
10 + 35 minutes

STORAGE
Make in advance and refrigerate for up to 3 days or freeze in single portions.

SERVE THIS WITH...
crusty roll
chunk of cheese or ham
Date & Pecan Brownie
  (see page 133)
fruit

HEALTH BENEFITS
Corn is a rich source of nutrients, such as energy-giving carbohydrates, fiber, potassium, iron, and vitamins A, B, and C.

If corn is in season, use the corn from 3–4 fresh cobs; if not, use canned.

1 tbsp. sunflower oil
1 large onion, chopped
1 carrot, chopped
2 potatoes, peeled and cubed
3–4 corn cobs, corn sliced off
  (optional)
1 bay leaf

3¾ cups gluten-free vegetable
  stock
14oz. can no-salt, no-sugar
  corn, drained (optional)
1¼ cups milk
salt
freshly ground black pepper

1 Heat the oil in a large saucepan and fry the onion, half-covered, 7 minutes until softened. Add the carrot, potatoes, fresh corn (if using), and bay leaf, and cook, half-covered, another 3 minutes.
2 Pour in the stock, bring to a boil, reduce the heat, and simmer 10 minutes. Add the canned corn (if using) and simmer a further 15 minutes, stirring occasionally.
3 Pour in the milk, gently heat through, then season to taste. Serve chunky, semi-chunky, or smooth, as wanted.

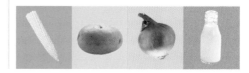

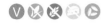

spicy carrot & lentil soup

This lightly spiced soup provides an impressive collection of nutrients. Red lentils are perfect for thickening soups because they eventually break down during cooking into a comforting puree.

1 tbsp. sunflower oil
1 large onion, chopped
1 stalk celery, finely chopped
4 carrots, thinly sliced
¾ cup split red lentils
1 tsp. ground cumin

1 tbsp. mild curry powder
5 cups gluten-free vegetable stock
salt
freshly ground black pepper

1 Heat the oil in a large saucepan and fry the onion over a medium-low heat 7 minutes, half-covered, until softened. Add the celery and carrots and cook another 3 minutes. Rinse the lentils.

2 Stir in the spices and lentils and cook, stirring, 1 minute, then pour in the stock. Bring to a boil then reduce the heat and simmer, half-covered, 35 minutes until the lentils are very soft and mushy. Occasionally skim off any foam created by the lentils during cooking.

3 Puree in a blender or using a hand blender and season to taste.

SERVES 4

PREPARATION + COOKING
15 + 50 minutes

STORAGE
Make in advance and refrigerate for up to 3 days or freeze in single portions.

SERVE THIS WITH...
wholewheat pita bread
Winter Fruit Salad (see page 122)

HEALTH BENEFITS
Sometimes known as Egyptian lentils, split red lentils are an excellent low-fat protein food, full of immune-supporting antioxidants.

SERVES 4

PREPARATION + COOKING
15 + 30 minutes

STORAGE
Make in advance and refrigerate
for up to 3 days or freeze in
single portions.

SERVE THIS WITH...
wholewheat bread
chunk of cheese or slices of ham
Banana & Blueberry Muffin
  (see page 132)
fruit

HEALTH BENEFITS
The orange flesh of the pumpkin
or squash provides plentiful
amounts of beta-carotene as
well as vitamins B, C and E,
magnesium, and potassium. Our
bodies are more able to make the
most of beta-carotene when it is
cooked with a little oil.

Ⓥ Ⓧ Ⓧ Ⓧ

hallowe'en soup

Pumpkin or squash makes a thick, creamy soup
with a touch of sweetness that goes down well
with children.

1 tbsp. olive oil
1 onion, chopped
1 carrot
1 stalk celery, chopped
¾ lb. peeled pumpkin or
  butternut squash,
  cut into chunks
1 bay leaf (optional)

1 tsp. dried mixed herbs
  (optional)
1 tbsp. curry powder (optional)
2 sprigs rosemary
5 cups gluten-free vegetable
  stock
salt
freshly ground black pepper

1 Heat the oil in a large saucepan and fry the onion
7 minutes, then add the carrot, celery, and pumpkin or
squash. Half-cover the pan and cook another 3 minutes.
2 Add the herbs (or curry powder for a spicy soup) and
stock and bring to a boil then reduce the heat and simmer,
half-covered, 20 minutes until the vegetables are tender.
3 Remove the bay leaf and rosemary. Puree in a blender or
using a hand blender. Season to taste.

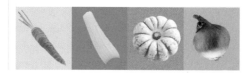

miso & tofu broth

Look out for packs of instant miso in supermarkets and health-food stores. They simply need the addition of hot water to make a simple savory stock and are an excellent base for a speedy Japanese-style soup.

2oz. fine egg noodles
1 sachet instant miso
    soup powder
½ carrot, cut into very thin strips
1 scallion, cut into
    thin strips
1 tsp. soy sauce
1 tsp. toasted sesame seeds

fingernail-size piece fresh
    ginger, peeled and cut into
    thin strips
4 (½in.) cubes soft tofu
sprinkling of nori flakes
    (optional)
pinch of dried chili flakes
    (optional)

1 Cook the noodles following the packet instructions; drain.
2 Rehydrate the instant miso soup powder in a saucepan, following the package instructions.
3 Add the cooked noodles, carrot, scallion, soy sauce, sesame seeds, ginger, tofu, nori flakes, and chili, if using, and heat through 1 minute.

SERVES 1

PREPARATION + COOKING
10 + 5 minutes

STORAGE
Make on the day.

SERVE THIS WITH...
Summer Pudding (see page 130)
fruit

HEALTH BENEFITS
Miso, which is made from a combination of cooked soybeans, rice, wheat, or barley that is left to ferment, is said to help eliminate toxins from the body.

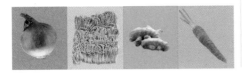

chunky italian soup

HEALTH BENEFITS
There's an element of truth in the adage that carrots help you see in the dark. Research has shown that eating just one carrot a day can help to improve night vision; this is because of its significant beta-carotene content. Chickpeas are high in zinc.

This nutritionally balanced soup contains carbohydrate, protein, fiber, vitamins, and minerals—in fact it's a complete meal in itself that will keep energy levels well sustained for the afternoon ahead.

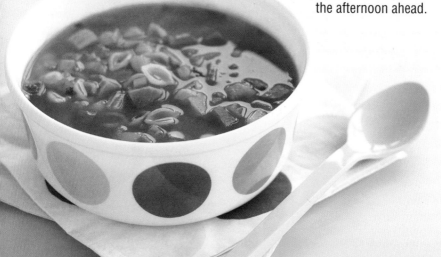

½ cup small pasta shapes such as conchigliette (small shells)
1 tbsp. olive oil
1 onion, chopped
1 stalk celery, chopped
1 large carrot, diced
1 tsp. dried oregano

2 bay leaves
5 cups vegetable stock
scant ½ cup passata (strained tomatoes)
scant 1 cup canned no-salt, no-sugar chickpeas, drained and rinsed

SERVES 4–6

PREPARATION + COOKING
15 + 30 minutes

STORAGE
Make in advance and refrigerate for up to 3 days or freeze in single portions.

SERVE THIS WITH...
chunk of cheese or slices of ham or sausage
Apple Flapjack (see page 126)
fruit

1 Cook the pasta following the instructions on the packet until al dente; drain, and rinse under cold running water.
2 Meanwhile, put the oil in a large saucepan and add the onion. Half-cover the pan and sauté the onion 7 minutes, stirring occasionally. Add the celery, carrot and herbs, and sauté another 3 minutes.
3 Pour in the stock and passata and add the chickpeas. Bring to a boil, then reduce the heat, and simmer, half-covered, 15 minutes. Add the pasta, stir, and cook another 5 minutes.

Chickpeas are low in fat and high in fiber. They are equally delicious hot or cold, and are very versatile.

 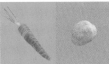 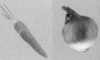

chicken noodle soup

SERVES 4

PREPARATION + COOKING
15 + 35 minutes

STORAGE
Make in advance and refrigerate for up to 3 days or freeze in single portions (unless the chicken was frozen).

SERVE THIS WITH…
Carrot Cake (see page 134)
fruit

HEALTH BENEFITS
A useful low-fat (as long as it is skinless) source of protein, chicken also provides selenium. This mineral is often missing in the diet and is a valuable immunity-boosting antioxidant.

Nurturing and sustaining, this is a great soup for a cold winter's day. For a vegetarian soup use vegetable stock and Quorn or extra veg.

½ cup fine egg noodles
1 tbsp. olive oil
1 onion, finely chopped
1 stalk celery, finely chopped
1 carrot, diced
1 bay leaf
7oz. skinless chicken breast, cut into bite-size pieces

5 cups chicken stock
2 tbsp. reduced-fat crème fraîche
1 tbsp. chopped flat-leaf parsley (optional)
salt
freshly ground black pepper

1 Cook the noodles following the package instructions until al dente; drain and rinse under cold running water.

2 Meanwhile, put the oil in a large saucepan and add the onion. Half-cover the pan and sauté the onion 7 minutes, stirring occasionally. Add the celery, carrot, and bay leaf, and sauté another 3 minutes.

3 Add the chicken and sauté 3–4 minutes, turning occasionally, until the chicken is golden all over.

4 Pour in the stock and bring to a boil, then reduce the heat and simmer 20 minutes until the chicken is cooked. Stir in the crème fraîche and cooked noodles and warm through. Season and add the parsley, if using.

ham & barley broth

A complete meal in a pot—this soup contains carbohydrate (barley) and protein (pancetta), plus a healthy amount of vegetables. Vegetarians can omit the ham and serve cheese on the side.

3½oz. pearl barley
1 tbsp. olive oil
1 large leek, finely sliced
1 large carrot, finely diced
3oz. pancetta or lean smoky
    bacon, diced

1 bay leaf
1 tsp. dried mixed herbs
5 cups wheat-free vegetable
    stock
salt
freshly ground black pepper

1 Soak the barley in cold water about 2 hours—this will help to speed up the cooking time. Drain and rinse.

2 Heat the olive oil in a large saucepan and fry the leek 5 minutes, then add the carrot, pancetta or bacon, and, barley and cook another 2 minutes.

3 Add the herbs and stock and bring to a boil. Reduce the heat and simmer, half-covered, 40–45 minutes, stirring occasionally, until the barley is tender. Season to taste.

SERVES 4

PREPARATION + COOKING
10 + 55 minutes + soaking

STORAGE
Make in advance and refrigerate for up to 3 days or freeze in single portions.

SERVE THIS WITH...
chunk of cheese
Roasted Red Bell Pepper
  Hummus (see page 28)
breadsticks
cereal bar
fruit

HEALTH BENEFITS
Believed to be the oldest cultivated grain, barley contains fiber, iron, calcium, and B vitamins. In traditional medicine, barley is thought to boost physical strength.

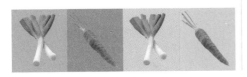

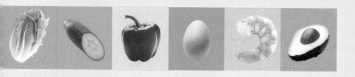

SANDWICHES & WRAPS

With such an abundance of different breads to choose from, there is no need to stick to the same type every day. Experiment with various varieties such as pita breads, flatbreads, bagels, rolls, ciabatta and baguettes, and breads made with different types of flour, such as sourdough and wholewheat. Cut sliced bread into interesting shapes using cookie cutters or roll it to create spirals. Wraps are a great idea for lunchboxes: cover soft flour tortilla wraps with all manner of fillings, then roll them up. Or why not try using rice paper wraps, lettuce leaves, or even an omelet as a wrap—an altogether more interesting variation on bread?

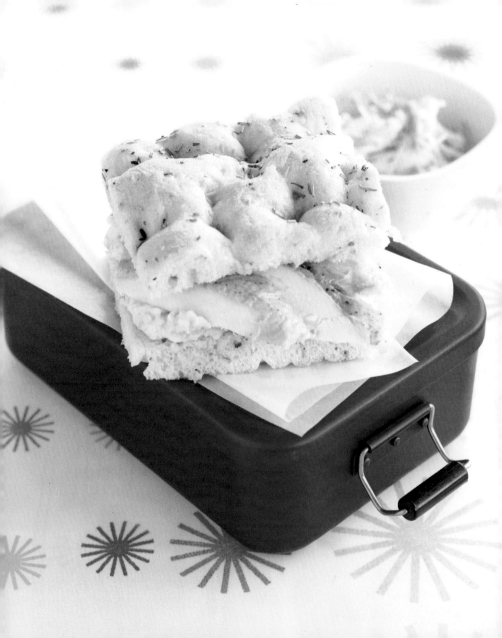

nut butter & banana bagel

The beauty of homemade nut butter is that you can choose your favorite combination of nuts and use no additives. If you can't find a cold-pressed oil that includes a blend of omega fats, use sunflower or canola oil instead.

SERVES ABOUT 8

PREPARATION + COOKING
15 + 5 minutes

STORAGE
Make the nut butter in advance and refrigerate for up to 2 weeks. Assemble on the day.

SERVE THIS WITH...
Cheesy Celery Stalks
  (see page 22)
carrot sticks
Chewy Date Bar (see page 127)
fruit

HEALTH BENEFITS
Cashew nuts are high in iron, zinc, magnesium, selenium, and B vitamins—a great immune-boosting combination.

1 sesame seed bagel
½ small banana, thinly sliced

4–5 tbsp. omega-blend or
  sunflower or canola oil
½ tsp. salt

Nut butter:
½ cup unsalted cashew nuts
½ cup unsalted peanuts

1 Lightly toast the nuts in a dry skillet over medium-low heat 4–5 minutes, turning regularly, until the nuts smell slightly toasted and are a light golden color.
2 Let the nuts cool and rub off the brown papery skin covering the peanuts, if necessary. Put the nuts, oil, and salt in a food processor and blend to a coarse paste. Place the nut butter in a lidded jar in the refrigerator.
3 Cut the bagel in half and spread the nut butter over one half. Arrange the slices of banana on top and cover with the other bagel half.

cream cheese & date bagel

Low-fat cream cheese is a perfect base for many different flavorings, both sweet and savory. Its smooth, creamy texture also means that there is no need for butter.

2 ready-to-eat dried dates	1 cinnamon bagel
1 tbsp. low-fat cream cheese	

1 Snip the dates into small pieces using scissors. Mix the dates into the cream cheese.
2 Cut the bagel in half and spread the date and cream cheese filling in the middle.

SERVES 1

PREPARATION
5 minutes

STORAGE
Make on the day.

SERVE THIS WITH...
Apple Coleslaw (see page 76)
cookie
fruit

HEALTH BENEFITS
Dates are a rich source of iron, which is essential for the formation of red blood cells and therefore beneficial to circulation.

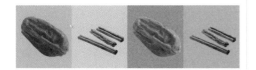

cheese, apple & chutney bun

Cheddar cheese and apple are a great combo. The homemade fresh fruity chutney is delicious, but you could use a little mayonnaise instead.

2–3 tbsp. grated mature
cheddar cheese
½ small apple, cored
and grated
1 seeded wholewheat bun

Chutney:
4 tomatoes, roughly chopped
1 large apple, peeled, cored,
and roughly chopped
1 onion, grated
5 tbsp. white wine vinegar
¼ cup sugar

1 Put all the chutney ingredients in a saucepan. Bring to a boil, then reduce the heat, cover, and simmer 5 minutes. Uncover the pan then cook a further 20 minutes. Let cool and spoon into a lidded jar.
2 Mix together the cheese, apple, and 2 teaspoons of chutney. Cut the bun in half and add the filling.

mystery roll

Children will love this hollowed-out crusty roll with its hidden filling. This typical Provençal "sandwich," otherwise known as *pan bagnat*, is best made the day before to allow the flavors to mingle. You could use tuna, chicken, or roasted vegetables instead of the cheese.

1 crusty roll
olive oil, for brushing
1–2 tbsp. pesto
1 small clove garlic, crushed
  (optional)

4 slices mozzarella cheese
1 tomato, seeded and sliced
small handful of baby
  spinach leaves

1 Slice off the top of the roll to make a lid and pull out the soft inside, leaving the crust intact. Lightly brush the inside of the roll with olive oil.

2 Put the bread in a food processor and pulse until you have breadcrumbs. Transfer to a bowl and stir in sufficient pesto to flavor the breadcrumbs without making them soggy, and the garlic, if using.

3 Spoon a layer of the breadcrumbs into the roll. Add a layer of mozzarella, tomato, and spinach followed by the rest of the breadcrumbs and the remaining mozzarella, tomato, and spinach. Place the lid on top and wrap tightly. Press down lightly.

SERVES 1

PREPARATION
15 minutes

STORAGE
Make the day before and refrigerate overnight.

SERVE THIS WITH...
Savory Spicy Popcorn
  (see page 21)
celery stalks
Cinnamon-spiced Apples
  (see page 120)

HEALTH BENEFITS
Spinach is one of the most nutritious of salad leaves and has a milder, less bitter flavor when uncooked, which also means it is richer in vitamins C and B. It also provides significant amounts of the eye-protecting antioxidant lutein.

bbq tofu baguette

The sweet, sticky marinade gives the tofu a rich, golden color and smoky BBQ taste. Griddling the tofu also enhances its BBQ flavor, although you could fry it in a little oil or roast in the oven 20 minutes instead.

SERVES 1 (TOFU SERVES 2)

PREPARATION + COOKING
10 + 8 minutes + marinating

STORAGE
Prepare and cook the tofu in advance and refrigerate for up to 3 days. Assemble on the day.

SERVE THIS WITH...
cucumber and celery sticks
Strawberry Crunch Cup
  (see page 124)
fruit

HEALTH BENEFITS
Tofu is the richest non-dairy source of calcium—in fact, a 3½oz. serving provides about half the daily allowance of calcium required by the 11–24 years age group.

olive oil, for brushing
4½oz. firm tofu, patted dry and
    cut into 4 long slices
1 small baguette
1 lettuce leaf, shredded
1 tomato, seeded and
    thinly sliced

Marinade:
1 tbsp. honey or
    sweet chili sauce
1 tbsp. tomato ketchup
1 tbsp. soy sauce
¼ tsp. smoked paprika
    (optional)

1 In a shallow dish, mix together the ingredients for the marinade. Place the tofu slices in the dish with the marinade. Spoon the marinade over the tofu so it is well coated. Let marinate for at least 1 hour or overnight.
2 Generously brush a griddle pan with olive oil, then heat until hot. Carefully put the tofu slices in the pan and cook 4 minutes on each side until golden, occasionally spooning over more of the marinade.
3 Slice the baguette lengthwise and open it out. Place two of the tofu slices in the baguette and top with the lettuce and tomato. Close up the baguette and press down lightly.

egg & bacon roll

You can't beat egg and bacon as a flavor combination, but this version also benefits from the tomato and super-healthy alfalfa sprouts.

1 slice bacon
1 free-range egg
1 ciabatta roll

½ tomato, seeded
few alfalfa sprouts
freshly ground black pepper

1 Heat the broiler to medium-high and line the broiler pan with foil. Broil the bacon until crisp, then let cool.
2 Meanwhile, boil the egg about 6 minutes until the yolk is still very slightly runny. Hold the egg under cold running water until it is cool enough to handle.
3 Peel the egg, place in a bowl, and roughly chop. Cut the bacon into small pieces and stir into the egg. Season.
4 Cut the ciabatta roll in half. Squeeze the tomato half and rub it into one half of the ciabatta. Spoon the egg and bacon mixture over the top and sprinkle with a few alfalfa sprouts. Put the other half of the ciabatta on top.

SERVES 1

PREPARATION + COOKING
10 + 7 minutes

STORAGE
Make the filling the day before and refrigerate overnight. Assemble on the day. Keep chilled until ready to eat (see page 11).

SERVE THIS WITH...
Creamy Guacamole (see page 31) and crudités
Apple Flapjack (see page 126)
fruit

HEALTH BENEFITS
Combining foods can improve the absorption of nutrients. The iron uptake from the eggs and bacon can be enhanced by eating them with vitamin C-rich foods such as tomatoes and alfalfa. A glass of fresh orange juice will also be of benefit.

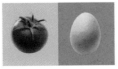

herrings on rye

This is best assembled at the time of eating, which means it's probably more suitable for older children. Store the herrings in a lidded jar then spoon them on to slices of rye bread. Herrings come in various marinades, including mustard, red onion, and sweet vinegar, so choose what you think will go down the best.

SERVES 1

PREPARATION
5 minutes

STORAGE
Make on the day. Keep chilled until ready to eat (see page 11).

SERVE THIS WITH...
sliced beet
vegetable chips
Banana & Blueberry Muffin
  (see page 132)
fruit

HEALTH BENEFITS
Herring is part of the oily fish family. There are literally hundreds of pieces of research that show the benefits of eating oily fish, from reducing blood pressure and cholesterol to improving brain power and concentration.

low-fat cream cheese,
  for spreading

2 slices rye bread
6 slices marinated herring

1 Spread the cream cheese over each slice of rye bread and sandwich with the cheesy sides in the middle.
2 Put the herrings in a jar with a lid. To eat, fork the herrings on to the bread or eat them separately straight from the container, if that is easier.

sardines & tomato on brown

Canned sardines are not only a convenient pantry essential, they're also healthy, versatile, and economical. If your child is anti-fish, try experimenting with the various different flavor options available.

4oz. can sardines in olive oil, drained
1 tomato, seeded and finely chopped
1 tsp. mayonnaise
½ tsp. grain or mild mustard
2 slices wholewheat bread (toasted if preferred)

1 Put the sardines in a bowl and mash with a fork. Add the tomato and mix with the sardines.
2 Mix together the mayonnaise and mustard, and spread over one slice of bread. Spoon on the sardines and tomato, and place the other slice of bread on top. Cut into triangles.

SERVES 1

PREPARATION
10 minutes

STORAGE
Make on the day. Keep chilled until ready to eat (see page 11).

SERVE THIS WITH...
carrot sticks
Soy-coated Nuts & Seeds (see page 20)
Summer Fruit Salad (see page 121)

HEALTH BENEFITS
All canned oily fish provide omega-3 fatty acids, although canned tuna has negligible amounts. Canned sardines have very soft bones that are barely distinguishable but are an excellent source of calcium.

cajun salmon & cucumber roll

SERVES 1

PREPARATION
5 minutes

STORAGE
Make on the day. Keep chilled
until ready to eat (see page 11).

SERVE THIS WITH...
avocado slices
Chewy Date Bar (see page 127)
grapes

HEALTH BENEFITS
Salmon provides rich amounts of
vitamin D, which is good for the
skin and valuable for people who
get little of this important vitamin
from sunlight.

Canned salmon sandwiches are reminiscent of days gone by, but a simple sprinkling of spices adds a new twist. Try to buy wild Alaskan salmon from sustainable sources.

¹/₃ cup canned salmon,
   skin removed
¼–½ tsp. mixed Cajun spices
squeeze of lemon juice

crusty brown roll
1 tsp. mayonnaise
5 slices cucumber

1 Spoon the salmon into a bowl and mix with the spices. Squeeze some lemon juice over the top.
2 Cut the roll in half and spread one side with the mayonnaise. Spoon the salmon on top, followed by the cucumber slices. Place the other half of the roll on top.

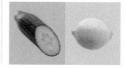

smoked salmon spirals

Simply by experimenting with different shapes and sizes, you can make a sandwich more interesting and fun. The lemon cream cheese adds a new twist to this classic filling.

1 tbsp. low-fat cream cheese
squeeze of lemon juice
1 slice wholewheat bread

1 slice white bread
slices of smoked salmon or trout
freshly ground black pepper

1 Mix the cream cheese with the lemon juice and season with pepper.
2 Cut the crusts off both slices of bread and spread the lemon cream cheese over one slice. Arrange a layer of fish on the bread and top with the remaining slice of bread.
3 Press down on the sandwich to flatten it slightly, then roll it up tightly into a cylinder shape. Wrap in plastic wrap until ready to slice. Cut the bread into ½-inch slices.

SERVES 1

PREPARATION
10 minutes

STORAGE
Make the day before and refrigerate overnight. Slice on the day. Keep chilled until ready to eat (see page 11).

SERVE THIS WITH...
Roasted Red Bell Pepper
  Hummus (see page 28)
carrot and cucumber sticks
fruit yogurt
raisins

HEALTH BENEFITS
Wholewheat flour provides more fiber, vitamins, and minerals than white flour, which loses much of its nutrients during processing— although it is now possible to buy white bread with similar nutrient levels to brown!

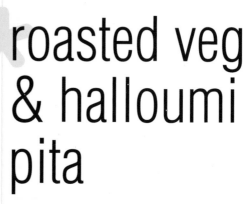

HEALTH BENEFITS
It is recommended that every day we eat a "rainbow" of different-colored fruit and vegetables. There's good reason for this, because each color provides a range of nutritious phytochemicals (plant nutrients), vitamins, and minerals.

roasted veg & halloumi pita

Vegetables when roasted seem to lose any trace of bitterness and take on a delicious caramelized sweetness; and they're just as good served cold as hot. Halloumi is a traditional Cypriot cheese that is at its best when griddled or fried quickly in a little oil.

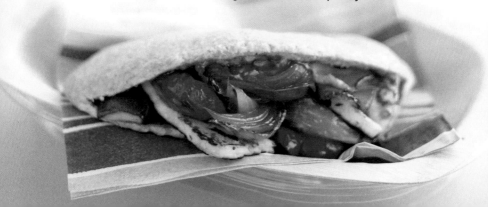

2½ tbsp. olive oil
1 tbsp. balsamic vinegar
1 small red bell pepper, seeded
   and cut into 8 slices
1 small zucchini,
   sliced lengthwise

1 small onion, cut into 8 wedges
2 tomatoes, halved
4 slices halloumi cheese,
   patted dry
2 wholewheat pita breads

SERVES 2

PREPARATION + COOKING
15 + 35 minutes

STORAGE
Cook the vegetables and
halloumi in advance and
refrigerate for up to 3 days.
Assemble on the day.

SERVE THIS WITH...
Soy-coated Nuts & Seeds
  (see page 20)
Mango Fool (see page 123)
fruit

1 Heat the oven to 400°F. Mix together 2 tablespoons of oil and balsamic vinegar in a shallow dish. Add the red bell pepper, zucchini, onion, and tomatoes, and turn the vegetables to coat them in the oil mixture.

2 Put the vegetables, except the tomatoes, in a roasting pan. Roast 20 minutes, turning occasionally, then add the tomatoes. Return the pan to the oven and cook another 10–15 minutes until the vegetables are tender and slightly blackened around the edges. Let cool.

3 Meanwhile, wipe the remaining oil over a griddle or skillet and heat until hot. Griddle or fry the halloumi a few minutes, turning once, until beginning to turn golden.

4 Slice each pita lengthwise, leaving each end intact, and open out to make a large pocket. Divide the vegetables and halloumi between the pitas and close to encase the filling.

The balsamic vinegar helps to caramelize the vegetables and adds a slight sweetness.

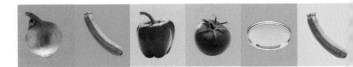

036

pipérade pita

Pipérade is a French Basque recipe based on scrambled eggs with bell pepper and tomatoes.

SERVES 1

PREPARATION + COOKING
10 + 4 minutes

STORAGE
Make on the day.

SERVE THIS WITH...
Carrot, Raisin & Pine nut Salad
(see page 77)
fresh berries and natural yogurt
dried apricots

HEALTH BENEFITS
Red bell pepper contains three
times the amount of vitamin C
and nine times the amount
of beta-carotene as its green
counterpart. It is also sweeter
in flavor, which tends to appeal
more to children.

1 tbsp. olive oil
1in. wide strip red bell pepper,
   diced
1 tomato, halved, seeded
   and diced
1 scallion, finely chopped

1 tbsp. milk
2 free-range eggs,
   lightly beaten
salt
freshly ground black pepper
wholewheat pita bread

1 Heat the oil in a skillet and fry the bell pepper gently
1 minute, then add the tomato and scallion and cook
another minute.
2 Mix the milk into the beaten eggs, season, and add to
the pan. Cook until the egg is scrambled (about 2 minutes),
stirring constantly with a wooden spoon to stop it sticking.
3 Warm the pita slightly to make opening it easier. Cut in
half crosswise then spoon the pipérade inside. Let cool
before wrapping.

kofta pita pockets

These lamb kofta are lightly spiced to give
them a Moroccan twist.

1 wholewheat pita	1 shallot, grated
1 tbsp. Roasted Eggplant Dip	1 clove garlic, crushed
(see page 32) or Tzatziki	¼ tsp. ground cinnamon
(see page 34)	1 tsp. ground cumin
mixed salad leaves	½ tsp. ground coriander
slices of tomato	olive oil, for brushing
	salt
Kofta:	freshly ground black pepper
½lb. lean ground lamb	

1 Put the lamb in a mixing bowl and break it up with a fork.
Add the shallot, garlic, and spices, season, and mix well.
2 Heat the broiler to medium. Shape the lamb mixture into
12 walnut-size balls. Line a broiler rack with foil and lightly
brush with oil. Broil the kofta 8–10 minutes, turning
occasionally, until golden. Let cool, then refrigerate.
3 Warm the pita slightly to make it easier to open out.
Cut in half crosswise to make two pockets, then spread a
little of your chosen dip (or you could use mayo, ketchup,
relish, mashed avocado, or hummus) inside each pocket.
4 Place a few lettuce leaves and slices of tomato in each
pocket, followed by two kofta, which can be left whole or
cut in half for easier eating.

MAKES 12 KOFTA (4 PER SERVING)

PREPARATION + COOKING
20 + 10 minutes

STORAGE
Make the kofta in advance and
refrigerate for up to 3 days
or freeze for up to 1 month.
Assemble on the day. Keep chilled
until ready to eat (see page 11).

SERVE THIS WITH…
Melon & Halloumi Salad
 (see page 78)
natural yogurt with honey
fruit

HEALTH BENEFITS
Spices have been prescribed
for their digestive properties for
hundreds of years. They also
have antibacterial qualities.

SERVES 1

PREPARATION
10 minutes

STORAGE
Make the day before and refrigerate. Keep chilled until ready to eat (see page 11).

SERVE THIS WITH...
Savory Spicy Popcorn
  (see page 21)
cherry tomatoes
Custard Tartlet (see page 135)
fruit

HEALTH BENEFITS
Like all meat products, you get what you pay for, so it really is worth splashing out on good-quality ham, which will have fewer additives.

ham roll-ups

A ham sandwich with a difference: it looks good, is easy to make, and takes the humble ham sandwich to a new dimension! You need a square loaf for the roll-ups to work.

2 thin slices square wholewheat loaf
a little butter
½ tsp. mild mustard or chutney
2 slices good-quality cooked ham, roughly the same size as the bread
2 long, thin sticks cucumber (the same length as each slice of bread), seeded

1 Remove the crusts from each slice of bread, then flatten them slightly by pressing down with your fingers. Mix the butter and mustard or chutney together in a bowl, then spread over the bread.

2 Lay a slice of ham on each slice of bread and place the cucumber diagonally across the ham.

3 Starting from one corner, roll each slice up tightly and place seam-side down on a board. Cut the roll-ups in half at an angle then wrap in plastic wrap to keep their shape.

tuna quesadilla

A great alternative to the usual tuna sandwich, this quesadilla can be made in two different ways: either folded into a pocket or cut into wedges.

2 slices mozzarella cheese	2 slices tomato
1 small soft flour tortilla	olive oil, for brushing
3–4 tbsp. canned tuna, drained	freshly ground black pepper

1 Place the mozzarella in the centre of the tortilla. Top with the tuna and tomato and fold in the sides of the tortilla to make a square pocket.

2 Brush a skillet with olive oil. Place the pocket seam-side down in the pan and fry over low heat about 3 minutes, turning once, until golden. Let cool before wrapping.

3 Alternatively, sandwich the filling between two tortillas, cook on both sides in a lightly oiled skillet until the cheese melts and the tortillas are slightly golden and crisp, then cut into wedges.

SERVES 1

PREPARATION + COOKING
5 + 3 minutes

STORAGE
Make on the day. Keep chilled until ready to eat (see page 11).

SERVE THIS WITH...
Pear & Ham Bundles
  (see page 24)
carrot sticks
Winter Fruit Salad (see page 122)

HEALTH BENEFITS
Mozzarella's fresh, mild flavor makes it popular with children, and as an added bonus it's low in fat.

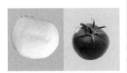

chicken tikka naan

Chicken is mild enough to absorb aromatic flavours, making it the perfect accompaniment to the curry sauce in this sandwich alternative.

SERVES 1

PREPARATION + COOKING
15 + 4 minutes + marinating

STORAGE
Prepare the chicken in advance and refrigerate for up to 3 days or freeze for up to 1 month (unless the chicken was frozen). Assemble on the day. Keep chilled until ready to eat (see page 11).

SERVE THIS WITH...
Soy-coated Nuts & Seeds
  (see page 20)
cucumber and celery sticks
Cinnamon-spiced Apples
  (see page 120)

HEALTH BENEFITS
Researchers have found that people who eat garlic on a regular basis are less likely to catch a cold than those who do not.

1 small skinless chicken
   breast, cut into strips
olive oil, for brushing
1 small naan bread
crisp salad leaves

Marinade:
3 tbsp. thick natural bio yogurt
1 clove garlic, crushed
1 tbsp. tikka curry paste

Yogurt dip:
1 tbsp. thick natural bio yogurt
1 tsp. chopped fresh mint

1 Mix together the ingredients for the marinade in a shallow dish. Add the chicken strips to the dish and spoon the marinade over until they are coated. Let marinate in the refrigerator 1 hour, or overnight if preferred.

2 Heat the broiler to medium-high and line the broiler pan with foil. Brush the foil with oil and place the marinated chicken on top. Broil 3–4 minutes on each side until cooked through. Let cool, then refrigerate.

3 Mix together the yogurt and mint. Split the naan in half, leaving one side attached. Place the chicken in the naan, followed by a few lettuce leaves, then spoon over the yogurt and mint and close up.

roast chicken & avocado focaccia

This is a great way to use up any leftovers from the Sunday roast, so feel free to swap the chicken for any type of roasted meat you have to hand—or indeed a nut roast would work equally well. You could add a few lettuce, watercress, or arugula leaves.

½ small avocado, pit removed	freshly ground black pepper
1 tsp. lemon juice	focaccia, about 4in. square
2 tsp. mayonnaise	(preferably the roasted red
salt	bell pepper variety)
	few slices roast chicken

1 Scoop the avocado out of its skin into a bowl. Mash with the lemon juice and mayonnaise. Season to taste.
2 Cut the focaccia in half crosswise. Spread the avocado over one half of the focaccia. Top with a few slices of chicken, then the other half of the focaccia.

SERVES 1

PREPARATION
10 minutes

STORAGE
Prepare the avocado the day before and refrigerate overnight. Assemble on the day.

SERVE THIS WITH...
Apple Coleslaw (see page 76)
Apricot Cookie (see page 136)
fruit

HEALTH BENEFITS
Avocados are almost a complete food, providing small amounts of protein, carbohydrate, and beneficial monounsaturated fats. They also contain the highest concentration of vitamin E of any fruit.

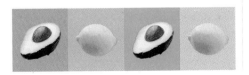

falafel & hummus lavash

PREPARATION
5 minutes

STORAGE
Make the falafel in advance and refrigerate for up to 3 days or freeze for up to 1 month. Assemble on the day.

SERVE THIS WITH...
Tabbouleh (see page 90)
Apricot & Cashew Nut Bar (see page 128)
fruit

HEALTH BENEFITS
Canned beans are a more convenient alternative to dried legumes, since they don't require lengthy soaking and cooking, but they still contain significant amounts of fiber, which is vital for a healthy digestive system.

Lavash is a Middle Eastern flatbread that makes an ideal wrap for all types of fillings. If you can't find one, then a soft flour tortilla will more than do. Or why not serve a falafel like a vegetarian burger in a small seeded bun?

1 lavash
1–2 tbsp. Roasted Red Bell Pepper Hummus (see page 28) or Creamy Guacamole (see page 31)

1 Falafel (see page 104)
few sprigs of arugula or watercress

1 Cut the lavash to the size of a small tortilla. Spread the hummus or guacamole over the lavash, then place the falafel in the center.

2 Arrange the arugula or watercress on top then fold in the bottom and sides to make a pocket, leaving the top open.

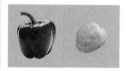

cool dogs

This healthier alternative to the hot dog is best made with good-quality, high-meat-content organic sausages and a soft wholewheat tortilla. The caramelized onions add a delicious sweet moistness but can be replaced with a dollop of good old ketchup, guacamole, or hummus, if preferred.

2 good-quality sausages or
   vegetarian alternative
2 tsp. olive oil
1 small onion, thinly sliced

1 tsp. balsamic vinegar
mild mustard, for spreading
1 soft wholewheat tortilla

1 Heat the broiler to medium-high and line the broiler pan with foil. Broil the sausages about 20 minutes, turning occasionally, until cooked through and golden.
2 Meanwhile, heat the oil in a skillet and fry the onion over medium-low heat about 10 minutes, stirring frequently. Pour in the balsamic vinegar, and cook the onions another 5–8 minutes until golden and glossy.
3 Spread a little mustard over the tortilla, then cut it in half. Divide the onions between the tortilla halves and top each one with a sausage. Fold in the rounded end of each tortilla half and roll up to encase the sausage.

SERVES 1

PREPARATION + COOKING
10 + 20 minutes

STORAGE
Cook in advance and refrigerate for up to 3 days. Assemble on the day. Keep chilled until ready to eat (see page 11).

SERVE THIS WITH...
Cheesy Celery Stalks
  (see page 22)
pretzels
Carrot Cake (see page 134)
fruit

HEALTH BENEFITS
Making onions a staple ingredient in your family's diet may greatly reduce the risk of several common cancers.

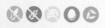

omelet wrap

HEALTH BENEFITS
Eggs provide valuable amounts of iron. A shortage of this mineral is relatively common and has been associated with delays in development and poor concentration.

However much we all like bread, it can become a bit dull if eaten every day. This recipe replaces a flour tortilla with an omelet wrap, which is rolled around crunchy, oriental-flavored vegetables. The shrimp are optional, and you could replace them with toasted sesame seeds, if you prefer.

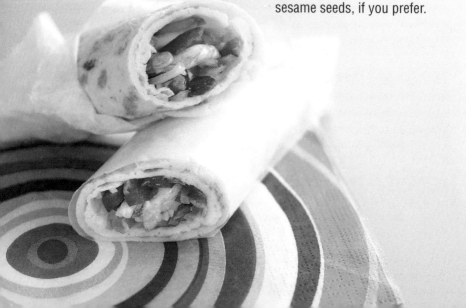

1 tsp. sunflower oil

2 free-range eggs,
  lightly beaten

1 scallion, cut into long, thin
  strips

¼ red bell pepper, seeded and
  cut into thin strips

2 sugar snap peas, sliced
  diagonally lengthwise

½ cup small cooked shrimp
  (optional)

½in. piece fresh ginger, peeled
  and grated

¼ tsp. toasted sesame oil

1 tsp. tamari (wheat-free
  soy sauce)

SERVES 1

PREPARATION + COOKING
10 + 3 minutes

STORAGE
Make the omelet the day before,
wrap and keep flat in the
refrigerator overnight. Assemble
on the day.

SERVE THIS WITH...
rice cakes
Apricot & Cashew Nut Bar
  (see page 128)
fruit

1 Heat the oil in a skillet. Pour the beaten egg into the pan
and swirl it around so that it covers the bottom. When the
egg begins to set, draw the edges toward the center using
a wooden spoon, allowing the raw egg to run into the
space. Cook about 2 minutes until the egg is set. Slide the
omelet onto a plate and let cool.

2 Put the scallion, red bell pepper, sugar snap peas,
shrimp, if using, and ginger in a bowl. Pour the sesame
oil and tamari over them and toss until they are coated.

3 Arrange the vegetables and shrimp down the center of
the omelet, then roll up, and cut in half.

Tamari, a by-
product of miso
is a type of soy
sauce suitable for
glucose-intolerant
people.

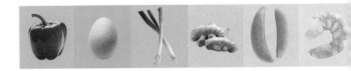

oriental beef wrap

A wrap with a difference—a crisp lettuce leaf rather than a tortilla encases this Chinese beef.

SERVES 1

PREPARATION + COOKING
10 + 2 minutes

STORAGE
Make the stir-fry the day before and refrigerate overnight. Strain off any liquid and assemble on the day. Keep chilled until ready to eat (see page 17).

SERVE THIS WITH...
Chinese Noodle Salad
(see page 85)
natural yogurt with honey
lychees

HEALTH BENEFITS
Red meat is one of the best sources of easily absorbed iron. Make sure you buy good-quality, lean, organic meat.

2 tsp. sesame oil
1 clove garlic, chopped
few slivers fresh ginger
3½oz. lean beef,
    cut into strips
2 tsp. tamari (wheat-free
    soy sauce)
1 tbsp. orange juice

2 iceberg lettuce leaves
1 scallion, shredded
2in. piece cucumber, seeded
    and cut into strips
¼ red bell pepper, seeded and
    cut into strips
cilantro leaves (optional)
freshly ground black pepper

1 Heat a wok over high heat and add the sesame oil, garlic, ginger, and beef, then stir-fry 1 minute. Add the tamari and orange juice, and stir-fry another minute until the liquid has reduced and thickened. Let cool.

2 Open out the lettuce leaves and divide the beef between them, spooning it down one half of each leaf. Top with the scallion, cucumber, bell pepper, and cilantro, if using.

3 Season and roll each leaf up to make a parcel. Cut each roll in half diagonally.

rice paper rolls

These rolls use pork, but you could use any
leftover roast meat or the beef stir-fry opposite.

½in. piece fresh ginger, peeled
and grated
1 tbsp. tamari (wheat-free
soy sauce), plus extra
for dipping
1 tsp. sesame oil
4 scallions, shredded
1 carrot, cut into matchsticks

½ yellow bell pepper, seeded
and cut into thin strips
20 medium rice paper wrappers
5 tbsp. gluten-free hoisin sauce
2oz. rice vermicelli noodles,
cooked
14oz. roast pork, cut into long,
thin strips

1 Mix together the ginger, tamari, and sesame oil in a bowl.
Add the scallions, carrot, and bell pepper and turn to coat.
2 Fill a heatproof bowl with just-boiled water. Put two rice
paper wrappers on top of one another and soak in the
water 20 seconds or until they are pliable and opaque.
Carefully remove using a spatula (they are very delicate),
drain for a second, and place flat on a plate.
3 Spread a teaspoonful of hoisin sauce over a wrapper,
then top with a small bundle of noodles, a few strips of
pork, and a few strips of scallion, carrot, and bell pepper.
4 Roll the wrapper around the filling, folding in the edges
to seal. Repeat using the remaining wrappers and filling
ingredients. Serve with a little cup of tamari to dip into.

MAKES 10

PREPARATION + COOKING
20 + 2 minutes

STORAGE
Make in advance and refrigerate
for up to 3 days or freeze for up
to 1 month. Keep chilled until
ready to eat (see page 17).

SERVE THIS WITH...
Soy-coated Nuts & Seeds
(see page 20)
cookie
fruit

HEALTH BENEFITS
Rice paper wrappers are ideal for
those who are allergic to wheat
or are gluten-intolerant.

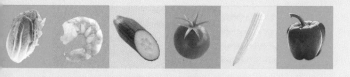

SALADS

The secret of the success of a lunchbox salad is to keep it cool, fresh, and crisp, and certain salads, such as those made with pasta, beans, potatoes, and noodles, withstand being transported much better than others, being more robust than those containing delicate leaves. The latter are best dressed just before eating, so if possible pack a cup of dressing that can be poured over when needed. Many of the salads in this chapter are substantial enough to be a main meal, particularly those that contain a carbohydrate element, such as pasta or beans, along with protein such as meat, seafood, or cheese. Salads made with grains, meat, and seafood need to be kept cool, so store in an insulated lunchbox with an ice-pack or refrigerate, if possible.

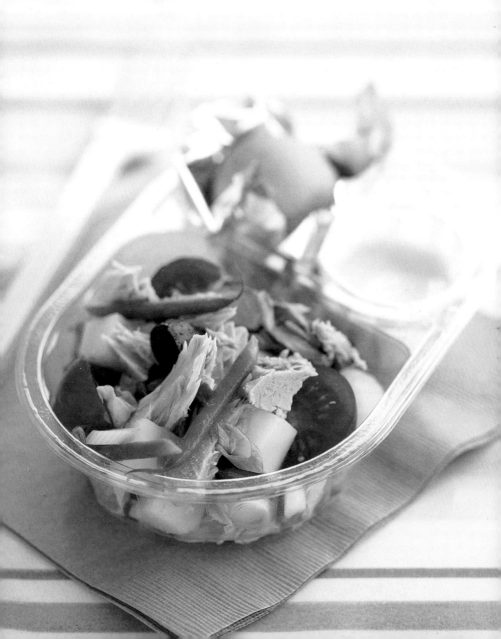

Ⓥ Ⓧ Ⓧ ⊗ Ⓞ

apple coleslaw

This is nothing like store-bought coleslaw, in which insipid vegetables come dripping in an additive-laden dressing. Crisp, crunchy, and packed with vitamins, this colorful salad will awaken the tastebuds. You could also sprinkle a handful of toasted seeds over the top.

SERVES 4

PREPARATION
10 minutes

STORAGE
Make in advance and refrigerate for up to 3 days.

SERVE THIS WITH...
Mini Tart (see page 102)
Apricot & Cashew Nut Bar
 (see page 128)
fruit

HEALTH BENEFITS
Cabbage when served raw is not only more nutritious than cooked, but is generally more acceptable to children, especially when finely shredded and lightly coated in a dressing. Numerous studies highlight cabbage's antiviral and antibacterial properties, and it is also believed to protect the body against certain forms of cancer.

4oz. red or white
    cabbage, grated
1 large carrot, grated
2 scallions, finely sliced
1 apple, cored and grated

Dressing:
1 tbsp. extra-virgin olive oil
1 tsp. lemon juice
1 tbsp. mayonnaise

1 Mix the cabbage, carrot, onions, and apple together in a bowl.
2 Whisk the oil and lemon juice together, then stir in the mayonnaise. Spoon the dressing over the salad and stir until combined.

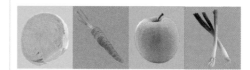

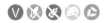

carrot, raisin & pine nut salad

Pine nuts are not nuts at all but the seeds of the Stone Pine tree, which is native to the Mediterranean region. They have the highest protein content of all seeds and nuts too.

1 heaped tbsp. pine nuts
1 large carrot, grated
1 heaped tbsp. raisins

Dressing:
1½ tbsp. extra-virgin olive oil
1 tsp. fresh lemon juice
¼ tsp. ground cumin

1 Put the pine nuts in a dry skillet and toast them over medium heat about 3 minutes, turning them occasionally, until slightly golden—take care as they can easily burn. Let the nuts cool, then place in a bowl with the carrot and raisins.
2 Mix together the dressing ingredients and pour over the salad before serving, turning until coated in the dressing.

SERVES 2

PREPARATION + COOKING
10 + 3 minutes

STORAGE
Make in advance and refrigerate for up to 3 days.

SERVE THIS WITH...
Chicken Strips with Satay Dip
  (see page 26)
wholewheat bread
Strawberry Crunch Cup
  (see page 124)

HEALTH BENEFITS
Raisins are a good source of potassium, which helps to regulate fluid levels in the body, along with energy-boosting iron.

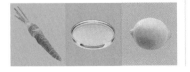

049

SERVES 1

PREPARATION + COOKING
5 + 6 minutes

STORAGE
Make the day before and
refrigerate overnight.

SERVE THIS WITH...
slices of pita bread
hummus
Date & Pecan Brownie
  (see page 133)
fruit

HEALTH BENEFITS
The vibrant orange color of
the cantaloupe melon comes
from lycopene, which can help
protect the skin from the sun's
UV rays. These melons also
contain beneficial amounts of
beta-carotene.

melon &
halloumi salad

Melon works particularly well with slightly salty
cheeses, such as halloumi, feta, or cheddar, or
meats such as crispy bacon, salami, or ham.

olive oil, for brushing
3 slices halloumi cheese,
  rinsed and patted dry
1 large wedge melon
mint leaves, chopped (optional)

Dressing:
1 tbsp. extra-virgin olive oil,
  plus extra for brushing
1 tsp. fresh lemon juice

1 Lightly brush a skillet with oil and heat. When the pan
is hot, put the halloumi in the pan and cook about 2–3
minutes on each side until light golden. Cut each slice
into quarters.
2 Remove the skin from the melon and cut it into chunks.
Combine with the halloumi.
3 Combine the dressing ingredients and pour over the
salad with some mint, if using, turning to coat the leaves.

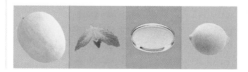

greek salad

Children like this chunky salad because all the ingredients are easily identifiable. It's also a salad that is easily transportable because it doesn't suffer when it gets swung around!

3oz. feta cheese, rinsed, patted
   dry, and cut into cubes
2 tomatoes, seeded and
   cut into chunks
4in. piece cucumber, cut into
   chunks
¼ small red onion, thinly sliced

8 black olives (optional)
1 tbsp. chopped mint or
   oregano leaves (optional)

Dressing:
2 tbsp. extra-virgin olive oil
2 tsp. fresh lemon juice

1 Put the feta in a bowl with the tomatoes, cucumber, red onion, and olives, if using.
2 Whisk together the oil and lemon juice and pour the dressing over the salad. Turn to coat the salad in the dressing and sprinkle with the mint or oregano, if using.

SERVES 2

PREPARATION
10 minutes

STORAGE
Make in advance and refrigerate for up to 2 days.

SERVE THIS WITH...
Roasted Eggplant Dip
  (see page 32)
toasted wedges of tortilla
Chewy Date Bar (see page 127)
fruit

HEALTH BENEFITS
A popular vegetable with the Greeks and Romans, cucumber is a good source of potassium and may help to relieve high blood pressure.

italian flag salad

Tricolore is a classic Italian salad that uses, patriotically, the same colors as its national flag. This version is able to withstand being carried about, but pack the avocado tightly in a container so that it is unable to slip around.

SERVES 1

PREPARATION
10 minutes

STORAGE
Prepare the tomato and mozzarella the day before, and refrigerate overnight. Assemble on the day.

SERVE THIS WITH...
Simple Mini Pizza (see page 100)
muffin
fruit

HEALTH BENEFITS
Avocados provide more than 25 essential nutrients, including vitamin E, B vitamins, folic acid, lutein, and fiber.

½ avocado, pit removed
lemon juice, for brushing
1 tomato, seeded and diced
1½oz. mozzarella cheese, cut into chunks
basil leaves (optional)

Dressing:
1 tbsp. extra-virgin olive oil
1 tsp. balsamic vinegar
freshly ground black pepper

1 Place the avocado in a plastic container that has a lid, making sure it is quite a tight fit, then brush a little lemon juice over the top to prevent it turning brown.
2 Arrange the tomato and mozzarella on top of the avocado, then sprinkle with a few basil leaves, if using.
3 Whisk together the dressing ingredients, store in a little lidded tub, and pour over the salad just before serving.

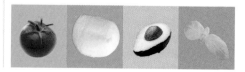

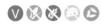

super salad

The word "super" is justly earned by this salad: sprouted beans and seeds are a nutritional powerhouse providing surprisingly high amounts of protein as well as vitamins and minerals. Bags of mixed sprouted beans are perfect for this: look for fresh, crisp sprouts.

3oz. mixed sprouted beans and
    seeds, such as chickpeas,
    alfalfa, mung beans, aduki
    beans, and lentils
4 radishes, thinly sliced
1 carrot, grated
½ small red onion, diced

Dressing:
1 tbsp. extra-virgin olive oil
2 tsp. sesame oil
1 tsp. grated fresh ginger
1 tsp. tamari (wheat-free
    soy sauce)
2 tsp. rice vinegar or lemon juice

1 Mix together the ingredients for the dressing; set aside.
2 Put the sprouted beans and seeds, radishes, carrot, and red onion in a bowl. Pour the dressing over the salad and turn to coat the ingredients in the dressing.

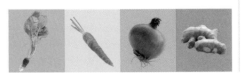

SERVES 2

PREPARATION
10 minutes

STORAGE
Make the day before and refrigerate overnight, with the dressing separate. Assemble on the day.

SERVE THIS WITH...
Tuna & Onion Tortilla
  (see page 111)
Custard Tartlet (see page 135)
fruit

HEALTH BENEFITS
Unlike most fruits and vegetables, whose nutrient levels start to diminish as soon as they are picked, the concentration of vitamins and minerals in sprouted beans and seeds continues to increase when sprouted. There are around 30 percent more B vitamins and 60 percent more vitamin C in the sprout than in the bean or seed in its original state.

*mixed bean salad

HEALTH BENEFITS
Foods rich in vitamin C, such as the apple and red bell pepper in this salad, will help your child's body to absorb the iron found in the legumes.

This salad is incredibly versatile: treat the beans as a base and add any favorite fruit, vegetables, nuts, seeds, or herbs you have to hand or that you know will go down well—the more colorful the better.

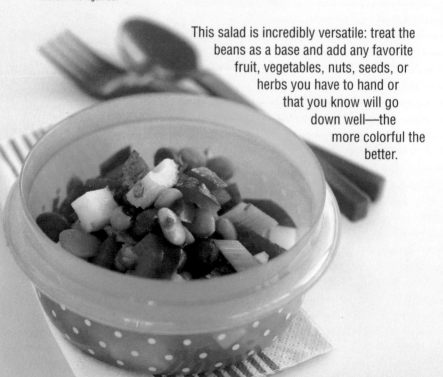

scant 3-cup can mixed beans,
drained and rinsed
1 red bell pepper, seeded
and diced
1 stalk celery, sliced
2 scallions, sliced
2 tbsp. chopped mint (optional)
1 apple, cored and diced
squeeze of lemon juice

Dressing:
2 tbsp. extra-virgin olive oil
2 tsp. white wine vinegar
½ tsp. English mustard powder
¼ tsp. sugar
salt
freshly ground black pepper

SERVES 4

PREPARATION
10 minutes

STORAGE
Make in advance and refrigerate
for up to 2 days.

SERVE THIS WITH...
Tandoori Chicken Drumstick
(see page 117) or
hard-boiled egg
mini pita bread
dried fruit

1 Mix together the dressing ingredients in a small bowl.
2 Put the beans in a serving bowl with the red bell pepper,
celery, scallions, and mint, if using.
3 Put the diced apple in another bowl, add the lemon juice,
toss to prevent the apple browning, then add to the salad.
4 Pour the dressing over the salad, then toss until
everything is mixed together.

**Aromatic mint
adds a fresh,
sweet flavor
to this salad
and also aids
digestion.**

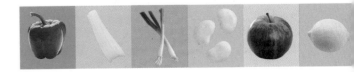

ham, bean & pineapple salad

This chunky, robust salad has a good mix of sweet and savory flavors. The fruit adds a delicious sweetness, which always goes down well with children, as well as a nutritional boost. Choose pineapple canned in natural juice rather than syrup.

1 cup canned pineapple,
   cut into chunks
5½oz. thickly cut
   good-quality ham, cubed
3½oz. canned cannellini beans,
   drained and rinsed

Dressing:
1 tbsp. natural juice from
   the pineapple
1½ tbsp. extra-virgin olive oil
2 tsp. white wine vinegar
½ tsp. Dijon mustard

1 Mix together the ingredients for the dressing.
2 Put the pineapple, ham, and beans in a bowl, then pour the dressing over the top. Toss the salad well to coat it thoroughly in the dressing.

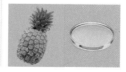

chinese noodle salad

Noodles are fun to eat and are just as good cold as hot. The oriental-style dressing not only has a delicious ginger and sesame flavor, but also prevents the noodles sticking together, which they can do when cold. For this reason it's best to pour the dressing over while they are warm.

heaped ½ cup medium egg
   noodles
1 carrot, cut into thin strips
2in. piece cucumber, seeded
   and cut into matchsticks
2 tomatoes, seeded and diced
2 scallions, finely sliced
3 tbsp. chopped cilantro or
   basil (optional)
1 tbsp. toasted sesame seeds

Dressing:
1 tbsp. olive oil
1 tsp. toasted sesame oil
1 tsp. soy sauce
1 tsp. grated fresh ginger
1 small clove garlic, crushed
1 tsp. lemon juice

1 Cook the noodles following the package instructions; drain and refresh under cold running water. Meanwhile, mix together the ingredients for the dressing. Pour it over the noodles and leave to cool.
2 Put the noodles, carrot, cucumber, tomatoes, scallions, and cilantro or basil, if using, in a bowl, then toss with your hands to mix. Sprinkle with the sesame seeds.

SERVES 2

PREPARATION + COOKING
15 + 5 minutes

STORAGE
Make in advance and refrigerate for up to 3 days.

SERVE THIS WITH...
Tofu Bites (see page 105)
fresh berries and natural yogurt

HEALTH BENEFITS
Noodles are low in fat. They are also an excellent source of selenium, thiamine, and folate, and a good source of niacin. Niacin and thiamine are both B vitamins; they work in tandem and are essential for the production of energy.

pesto pasta salad

SERVES 2

PREPARATION + COOKING
10 + 12 minutes

STORAGE
Make the day before and refrigerate overnight.

SERVE THIS WITH...
Pear & Ham Bundles
 (see page 24)
cookie
fruit

HEALTH BENEFITS
Surprisingly, frozen peas are often more nutritious than fresh. This is because freezing takes place soon after picking, before the vitamin values have fallen. Peas provide significant amounts of protein, vitamins B and C, and iron, making them a good choice for vegetarians.

Popular with kids, pesto makes a quick and easy dressing when mixed with mayonnaise. The small flowerets of broccoli add lots of goodness, but may not appeal to all children, so you can swap them for corn or bell pepper instead. New potatoes can replace the pasta.

1 cup farfalle pasta
6 small flowerets broccoli
2oz. frozen petits pois
2oz. mature cheddar cheese, cut
   into small chunks
salt

Dressing:
1 tbsp. mayonnaise
1–2 tbsp. pesto
squeeze of lemon juice
freshly ground black pepper

1 Bring a large saucepan of salted water to a boil. Add the pasta, stir, and cook following the package instructions until al dente. Drain well and refresh under cold water.
2 Meanwhile, steam the broccoli 4 minutes until only just tender—it should still be slightly crunchy. Add the peas about 1½ minutes before the end of the cooking time. Refresh the vegetables under cold running water.
3 Mix the dressing ingredients together, adding pesto to taste, and season with pepper. Put the pasta, vegetables, and cheddar in a bowl, and spoon the dressing over the top. Turn the salad with a spoon to coat it in the dressing.

shrimp pasta salad

A complete meal in a tub, this salad combines protein from the shrimp and carbohydrate from the pasta with lots of vitamins and minerals.

1 cup pasta shells
¼lb. cooked shelled small
   shrimp, defrosted if frozen
6 cherry tomatoes, quartered
crisp lettuce leaves, such as
   romaine, shredded

Dressing:
1 tbsp. mayonnaise
1 tsp. lemon juice
1 tbsp. tomato ketchup
2 drops Tabasco (optional)
salt
freshly ground black pepper

SERVES 2

PREPARATION + COOKING
10 + 12 minutes

STORAGE
Make in advance and refrigerate for up to 2 days. Assemble on the day. Keep chilled until ready to eat (see page 11).

SERVE THIS WITH...
Apricot & Cashew Nut Bar
  (see page 128)
fruit

HEALTH BENEFITS
Shrimp are rich in the antioxidant minerals selenium and zinc, which are good for the skin.

1 Bring a large saucepan of salted water to a boil. Add the pasta, stir and cook following the packet instructions until al dente. Drain well and refresh under cold water.
2 Put the shrimp and tomatoes in a bowl with the pasta and season with pepper.
3 Mix the dressing ingredients together and spoon over the salad. Turn the salad with a spoon to coat it well.
4 Serve the shrimp salad on a bed of shredded lettuce.

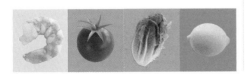

shrimp salad

SERVES 1

PREPARATION
10 minutes

STORAGE
Make the day before and refrigerate overnight. Assemble on the day. Keep chilled until ready to eat (see page 11).

SERVE THIS WITH...
crusty wholewheat bread
Apple Flapjack (see page 126)
fruit

HEALTH BENEFITS
Canned corn is a good source of readily usable fiber, as are beans; these help to keep the digestive system working efficiently.

This salad is arranged in distinct, colorful layers, which add to its appeal and flexibility. To keep the layers intact during the school day, pack the salad fairly tightly in an airtight tub.

1½oz. crisp lettuce leaves such as romaine, thickly sliced
2oz. canned beans of choice, drained and rinsed
1 carrot, finely grated
6 slices cucumber
3 tbsp. canned no-salt, no-sugar corn, drained
¼lb. cooked shelled shrimp

Dressing:
1 tbsp. extra-virgin olive oil
2 tsp. mayonnaise
½ clove garlic, crushed
1 tsp. lemon juice
salt
freshly ground black pepper

1 Mix together the ingredients for the dressing and keep in a small container until ready to use.

2 Arrange the salad ingredients in layers: salad leaves, beans, carrot, cucumber, corn, and shrimps. Spoon the dressing over the salad when ready to eat.

tuna niçoise

Keep the dressing separate and pour it over just before eating; refrigerate the remainder.

1 large Cos lettuce leaf, roughly sliced
2oz. cooked young green beans, halved
3 cooked small new potatoes, cut into cubes
3 cherry tomatoes, halved
1 scallion, sliced
6 pitted black olives, halved

¾ cup tuna, drained
1 hard-boiled free-range egg, shell left on

Dressing:
2 tbsp. extra-virgin olive oil
1 tsp. white wine vinegar
½ clove garlic, crushed
3 tbsp. mayonnaise

1 Arrange the Cos lettuce in the bottom of a tub. Place the green beans on top, then add the potatoes.
2 Next, put the tomatoes, scallion, and olives in the tub. Flake the tuna and place it on top. Leave the egg in its shell and wrap in foil.
3 Whisk together the ingredients for the dressing. Put one serving in a small container or drizzle it over the salad.
4 When ready to eat, peel the egg and serve with the salad.

SERVES 1 (DRESSING FOR 4)

PREPARATION
15 minutes

STORAGE
Prepare the ingredients the day before and refrigerate overnight. Assemble on the day. Keep chilled until ready to eat (see page 11).

SERVE THIS WITH...
Seeded Dough Balls (see page 139)
Mango Fool (see page 123)
fruit

HEALTH BENEFITS
Although canned tuna is not as rich in the beneficial omega-3 fatty acids as fresh tuna, it still provides useful amounts as well as B vitamins (vital for a healthy nervous system and energy metabolism) and selenium.

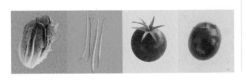

tabbouleh

This is a perfect salad for a lunchbox because it can withstand being carried around and tastes at its best when not over chilled. Bulgur wheat is most commonly used in this Middle Eastern salad, but you could also try brown rice, couscous, and protein-rich quinoa.

SERVES 2

PREPARATION + COOKING
10 + 15 minutes

STORAGE
Make in advance and refrigerate for up to 3 days.
Keep chilled until ready to eat (see page 11).

SERVE THIS WITH...
Falafel & Hummus Lavash (see page 68)
Apricot Cookie (see page 136)
fruit

HEALTH BENEFITS
Bulgur wheat has a light, nutty taste and is a better source of nutrients than white flour, as it contains more fiber and selenium.

$^1/_3$ cup bulgur wheat
3 small tomatoes, seeded and chopped
2 scallions, finely chopped
2in. piece cucumber, diced
3 tbsp. chopped mint
3 tbsp. chopped parsley

salt
freshly ground black pepper

Dressing:
1 tbsp. extra-virgin olive oil
2 tbsp. lemon juice

1 Put the bulgur wheat in a saucepan and cover it with cold water. Bring to a boil then reduce the heat, cover, and simmer 10–15 minutes until tender. Drain, if necessary, and let cool.
2 Put the bulgur wheat in a bowl with the tomatoes, scallions, cucumber, and herbs.
3 Mix together the olive oil and lemon juice and pour the dressing over the salad. Season to taste and turn the salad to coat it in the dressing.

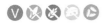

oriental rice salad

Vary this salad by adding different vegetables, meat, or fish to the rice and dressing base.

½ cup brown basmati rice
½ red bell pepper, seeded
   and diced
2 scallions, thinly sliced
3 baby corn, quartered
2 tbsp. toasted sunflower and
   sesame seeds

Dressing:
   2 tbsp. sunflower oil

1 tbsp. fresh apple juice
2 tsp. tamari (wheat-free
   soy sauce)
2 tsp. rice wine vinegar or
   white wine vinegar
½ tsp. Chinese five spice
   powder
1 tsp. honey
½–1 tsp. grated fresh ginger

1 Put the rice in a pan with plenty of salted water, bring to a boil then simmer 10 minutes, or until cooked. Drain, then rinse under cold running water until cold.

2 Put the cooked rice, red bell pepper, scallions, baby corn, and toasted seeds in a bowl.

3 Mix together the ingredients for the dressing, then pour over the salad, turning it gently until it is well coated.

SERVES 2

PREPARATION + COOKING
10 + 10 minutes

STORAGE
Make in advance and refrigerate for up to 2 days.
Keep chilled until ready to eat (see page 11).

SERVE THIS WITH...
Spring Roll (see page 113)
Winter Fruit Salad (see page 122)

HEALTH BENEFITS
Brown rice produces a gentler rise in blood sugar levels than white rice, potatoes, or bread, therefore keeping energy levels steady. Brown rice also has more nutrients than white and is higher in fiber and vitamin B1.

spicy bulgur salad with nectarines

HEALTH BENEFITS
Made from wheat berries, this light, nutty grain is a good source of dietary fiber and B vitamins as well as the immunity-boosting minerals iron and selenium.

Bulgur wheat is easy for children to eat and its mild flavor works well with this lightly spiced dressing. Add halloumi, mozzarella, or chicken to introduce some protein to the meal.

½ cup bulgur wheat
scant 2 cups vegetable stock
1 tbsp. olive oil
2 cloves garlic, chopped
1 tsp. ground cumin
1 tsp. ground coriander
½ tsp. ground cinnamon
1 ripe nectarine, halved, pit

removed, and sliced
3 tbsp. toasted pine nuts
(optional)
2 tbsp. chopped cilantro
(optional)
freshly ground black pepper

SERVES 4

PREPARATION + COOKING
10 + 18 minutes

STORAGE
Make in advance and refrigerate
for up to 3 days.
Keep chilled until ready to eat
(see page 11).

SERVE THIS WITH...
Cheesy Celery Stalks
(see page 22)
natural yogurt with honey
fruit

1 Put the bulgur wheat in a saucepan with the stock.
Bring to a boil, then reduce the heat, cover, and simmer
10–15 minutes until the stock is absorbed. Remove from
the heat and let the pan stand 5 minutes with the
lid on.
2 Meanwhile, heat the oil in a skillet and fry the garlic
1 minute, then add the spices, and cook another minute.
Remove from the heat, add the wheat, and stir to coat it
in the spices. Transfer to a bowl and let cool.
3 Stir in the nectarine, pine nuts, and cilantro, if using,
and season with pepper.

Fresh fruit in
salads adds
a valuable
nutritional boost
and a delicious
sweetness.

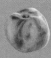

sausage & barley salad

SERVES 4

PREPARATION + COOKING
soaking + 15 + 20 minutes

STORAGE
Make in advance and refrigerate for up to 3 days or freeze for up to 1 month. Keep chilled until ready to eat (see page 17).

SERVE THIS WITH...
celery and carrot sticks
Banana & Blueberry Muffin
 (see page 132)
fruit

HEALTH BENEFITS
Barley has a mild, sweet flavor and chewy texture; its fiber content has been shown to help prevent constipation as well as heart disease and bowel disorders, including colon and rectal cancer.

This wholesome, robust salad is easy for children to eat. It's best to use organic sausages with a high meat content to avoid unnecessary additives and fillers.

heaped ½ cup pearl barley
6 good-quality sausages, or
   vegetarian alternative
2 tbsp. olive oil
2 cloves garlic, finely chopped

1 tsp. dried oregano
4 tbsp. canned tomatoes
salt
freshly ground black pepper

1 Soak the barley 6 hours or overnight; drain and rinse.
2 Heat the broiler to medium and line the broiler pan with foil. Broil the sausages, turning them occasionally, 20 minutes until cooked through and browned. Let cool.
3 Meanwhile, heat the oil in a skillet and fry the garlic 1 minute, stirring. Add the oregano, tomatoes, and barley and cook 10 minutes, stirring occasionally. Remove from the heat and let cool.
4 Slice the sausages and stir into the barley mixture.

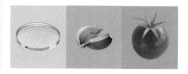

spicy sweet potatoes

These are a good introduction to curry flavors for kids who may be reluctant to try spicy foods. The dressing is also delicious with shrimp or chunks of poached chicken, or with a hard-boiled egg.

10oz. orange-fleshed sweet
 potato, peeled and cut into
 bite-size chunks
1 stalk celery, thinly sliced

Dressing:
1 tbsp. low-fat natural
 bio yogurt
¾ tsp. curry powder
1 tsp. smooth mango chutney
squeeze of lemon juice

1 Cook the sweet potato in plenty of boiling water about 8–10 minutes until tender. Drain and refresh the potato under cold running water to stop it cooking any further.
2 Meanwhile, mix the dressing ingredients in a bowl.
3 Put the potato and celery in a bowl, spoon the dressing on top, and turn the salad with a spoon to coat it well.

SERVES 2

PREPARATION + COOKING
10 + 10 minutes

STORAGE
Make in advance and refrigerate for up to 3 days.

SERVE THIS WITH...
Tandoori Chicken Drumstick
 (see page 117)
cucumber sticks
Chewy Date Bar (see page 127)
fruit

HEALTH BENEFITS
Containing far more vitamins than ordinary potatoes, sweet potatoes are a good source of iron, beta-carotene, and vitamin C and are the only low-fat food with a significant vitamin E content.

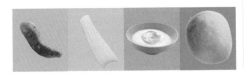

smoked mackerel, apple & potato salad

Mackerel is a much underrated oily fish, being healthy, cheap, and versatile. When smoked, it makes a protein-rich addition to a salad that works best with a slightly creamy dressing.

SERVES 2

PREPARATION + COOKING
15 + 12 minutes

STORAGE
Make the day before and refrigerate overnight. Assemble on the day. Keep chilled until ready to eat (see page 11).

SERVE THIS WITH...
Cheese Scones (see page 138)
cookie
fruit

HEALTH BENEFITS
Mackerel contains significant amounts of omega-3 fatty acids, which are vital for children's developing brains, eyes, skin, and nervous system.

9oz. new potatoes, scrubbed and halved if large
3oz. smoked mackerel fillets (or salmon or trout)
1 small red apple, cored and diced
2 stalks celery, finely chopped

Dressing:
1½ tbsp. mayonnaise
1 tbsp. extra-virgin olive oil
2 tsp. creamed horseradish
1 tsp. lemon juice, plus a little extra for the apple

1 Cook the potatoes in a pan of boiling water about 12 minutes until tender; drain and set aside to cool.
2 Meanwhile, mix together the ingredients for the dressing with 1 tablespoon of water until smooth and creamy.
3 Peel the skin off the mackerel and break into large chunks. Toss the apple in a little lemon juice to prevent it turning brown. Put the apple in a bowl with the mackerel, potatoes, and celery.
4 Spoon the dressing over the top. Turn the salad until it is coated in the dressing.

chicken caesar salad

This is a Caesar salad with a difference: the dressing has been adapted to make it more child-friendly and it also contains new potatoes, making it a nutritionally balanced lunch.

9oz. new potatoes, scrubbed, and halved if large
2 tsp. olive oil
5½oz. skinless chicken breast, cut into large bite-size pieces
2 romaine lettuce leaves, shredded
2 tomatoes, seeded and diced

Dressing:
1½ tbsp. mayonnaise
1½ tbsp. extra-virgin olive oil
2 tsp. lemon juice
1 small clove garlic, crushed
½ tsp. Dijon mustard
¼ tsp. gluten-free Worcestershire sauce
2 tbsp. finely grated Parmesan cheeese

1 Cook the potatoes in plenty of boiling water about 12 minutes until tender; drain and set aside to cool.
2 Meanwhile, heat the olive oil in a skillet and fry the chicken 5–6 minutes, turning occasionally, until golden and cooked through. Let cool.
3 Put the dressing ingredients in a blender and process until smooth and creamy.
4 Put the romaine lettuce in a bowl and add the potatoes, tomatoes, and chicken. Spoon over enough of the dressing to coat the salad.

SERVES 2

PREPARATION + COOKING
15 + 12 minutes

STORAGE
Make the day before and refrigerate overnight. Assemble on the day. Keep chilled until ready to eat (see page 11). The remaining dressing will keep in the refrigerator for up to 1 week.

SERVE THIS WITH…
a handful of walnuts or pretzels
Carrot Cake (see page 134)
fruit

HEALTH BENEFITS
Potatoes are a popular starchy carbohydrate and contain a higher concentration of vitamins and minerals if the skin is left on.

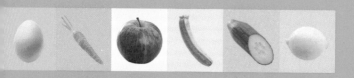

SAVORY BITES

Tired of sandwiches? Then this diverse selection of recipes should encourage you to ring the changes. Inspired by some of the cuisines of the world, there's a wide variety to choose from, including Italian Calzone and Simple Mini Pizzas, Spanish Tuna & Onion Tortilla, Chinese Spring Rolls, Japanese Sushi Cones, Middle Eastern Falafel, and Indian Tandoori Chicken Drumsticks. Most of the recipes take a little more preparation than a sandwich but all keep well and can be made in advance then chilled or frozen for convenience. Importantly, the recipes have been chosen to withstand being transported in a lunchbox and simply need the addition of vegetable sticks and salad to make them into a complete meal to sustain your child until dinner time.

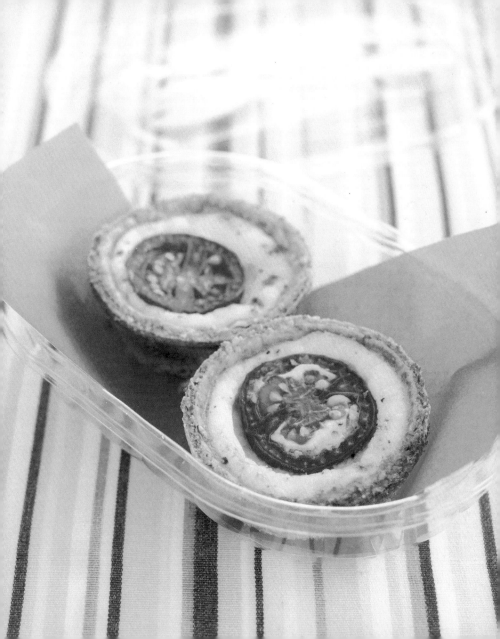

simple mini pizzas

MAKES 6

PREPARATION + COOKING
20 + 25 minutes

STORAGE
Make the day before and refrigerate overnight. The dough and sauce can be frozen separately for up to 1 month.

SERVE THIS WITH...
carrot and red bell pepper sticks
Mango Fool (see page 123)
fruit

HEALTH BENEFITS
Cheese provides valuable amounts of protein and calcium, essential for growing bones and teeth. However, cheddar is high in saturated fat so try to eat in moderate amounts and choose a mature cheese rather than a mild one, because its strong flavor means that you can use less.

The dough for these pizzas is made without yeast, which greatly speeds up preparation time.

1 tbsp. olive oil
²/₃ cup passata (strained tomatoes)
2 tsp. tomato paste
½ tsp. dried oregano
5½oz. ball mozzarella cheese, drained and sliced
2oz. mature cheddar cheese, grated

Dough:
1½ cups white self-rising flour, plus extra for dusting
¾ cup wholewheat self-rising flour
½ tsp. salt
²/₃ cup half-fat milk
4 tbsp. olive oil

1 Heat the oven to 400°F. Heat the oil in a saucepan and add the passata, tomato paste, and oregano; stir and bring to a boil. Half-cover and simmer 10 minutes, stirring occasionally, until reduced.

2 Sift the flours and salt into a mixing bowl, adding any bran left in the sifter. Make a well in the center and pour in the milk and oil. Mix with a fork until the ingredients start to come together into a dough (adding a little more milk if dry). Tip the dough out on to a floured work surface and knead briefly until it forms a smooth ball.

3 Divide into six pieces, roll into balls, then flatten into circles. Place on floured baking sheets. Divide the tomato sauce and cheeses among them. Bake 10 minutes.

calzone

This portable pizza has its filling safely inside.

1 tbsp. olive oil
1 onion, chopped
2 cloves garlic, chopped
1 large carrot, diced
1 small red bell pepper, seeded
and diced
9oz. vegetarian meat crumbles
1¾ cups passata (strained
tomatoes)
1 tsp. dried oregano
2 tbsp. tomato ketchup
freshly ground black pepper

4oz. mozzarella cheese, cut
into small pieces

Dough:
3 cups white self-rising flour,
plus extra for dusting
1½ cups wholewheat self-rising
flour
1 tsp. salt
1¹/₃ cups half-fat milk
8 tbsp. olive oil

MAKES 8

PREPARATION + COOKING
30 + 40 minutes

STORAGE
Make the day before and
refrigerate overnight.

SERVE THIS WITH...
Italian Flag Salad (see page 80)
grapes

HEALTH BENEFITS
Olive oil has a higher
concentration of
monounsaturated fat than any
other oil and has a protective
role in preventing heart disease.

1 Heat the oven to 400°F. Heat the oil in a saucepan and fry the onion 8 minutes, then stir in the other vegetables and cook another 3 minutes. Stir in the remaining ingredients and bring to a boil. Simmer 15 minutes until reduced. Season well and let cool.

2 Make the dough (see Simple Mini Pizzas, opposite), then divide into eight. Roll into thin disks about 4½ inches in diameter and divide the sauce and cheese among them.

3 Fold the disks in half, press the edges together, and crimp to seal. Prick the top with a fork. Place on floured baking sheets and bake 10–12 minutes until golden.

690

(V) (O)

mini tarts

Small tarts survive better in a lunchbox than individual slices, which are prone to breaking up.

MAKES 8

PREPARATION + COOKING
25 + 22 minutes + chilling

STORAGE
Make in advance and refrigerate for up to 1 week or freeze for up to 1 month.

SERVE THIS WITH...
carrot and cucumber sticks
Super Salad (see page 81)
Winter Fruit Salad (see page 122)

HEALTH BENEFITS
Both nutritious and convenient, eggs are now available that are fortified with omega-3 fatty acids, which benefit the immune system, skin, brain, and eyes.

²/₃ cup milk
4 free-range eggs, lightly beaten
2½oz. mature cheddar cheese, grated
1 tomato, sliced into 8 circles
salt
freshly ground black pepper

Dough:
1¹/₃ cups wholewheat plain flour
3½oz. cold unsalted butter, cut into small pieces
pinch of salt

1 Sift the flour into a bowl, adding any bran left in the sifter. Rub the butter into the flour using your fingertips until it forms breadcrumbs. Pour in 2 tablespoons of iced water and stir with a fork, then your hands, until it forms a ball. Wrap the dough in plastic wrap and chill 30 minutes.
2 Grease an eight-cup deep muffin pan. Roll out the dough on a floured surface and use to line the holes, leaving the dough slightly high at the top. Heat the oven to 400°F. Chill the dough shells 15 minutes.
3 Bake the dough shells 6 minutes then remove from the oven. Whisk the milk and eggs together and season. Sprinkle the cheese into the shells, add the egg mixture and a slice of tomato, and bake 15 minutes until set.
4 Cool slightly before removing with a palette knife.

ham & egg pies

These simple pies use ham as a base instead of pastry, keeping fat levels down and making them very quick and easy to make. Use a good-quality ham with high-meat, low-water content.

olive oil, for brushing
4 thin slices good-quality ham

4 free-range eggs

1 Heat the oven to 375°F. Lightly brush four cups of a deep muffin pan with oil.

2 Arrange a slice of ham in each cup, overlapping the sides where necessary. Carefully trim the top of the ham slices to make them even but leaving the ham slightly above the edge of the tin.

3 Crack an egg into a bowl, then drop it into a ham-lined hollow; repeat with the remaining eggs. Bake 10–12 minutes until the eggs are set.

4 Let cool slightly, then lift out the "pies" with a palette knife. Let cool completely.

MAKES 4

PREPARATION + COOKING
15 + 12 minutes

STORAGE
Make in advance and refrigerate for up to 3 days. Keep chilled until ready to eat (see page 11).

SERVE THIS WITH...
Tabbouleh (see page 90)
Carrot Cake (see page 134)
fruit

HEALTH BENEFITS
Eggs are rich in brain-boosting choline, which is used to produce the neurotransmitter acetylcholine, which is shown to aid memory.

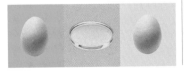

falafel

This is a great way to encourage your child to eat beans—other than the baked variety that is! Serve the falafel wrapped in a flatbread (see page 68) or on their own with a hummus dip.

MAKES 12

PREPARATION + COOKING
15 + 20 minutes + chilling

STORAGE
Make in advance and refrigerate for up to 5 days or freeze for up to 1 month.

SERVE THIS WITH...
Falafel & Hummus Lavash (see page 68) or Spicy Bulgur Salad with Nectarines (see page 92) Apricot Cookie (see page 136) fruit

HEALTH BENEFITS
A combination of protein provided by the chickpeas and carbohydrate from the flatbread has been shown in tests to help students perform better in exams and to help memory recall.

scant 3-cup can no-salt, no-sugar chickpeas, drained and rinsed
3 scallions, finely chopped
2 cloves garlic, crushed
1 tsp. ground cumin
1 tsp. ground coriander

1–2 tbsp. chopped mint (optional)
1 small free-range egg, lightly beaten
salt
freshly ground black pepper
all-purpose flour, for dusting
sunflower oil, for frying

1 Put the chickpeas, scallions, garlic, cumin, coriander, and mint, if using, in a food processor and pulse until the chickpeas are roughly chopped. Add the egg and seasoning and blend until the mixture forms a coarse paste. Chill 1 hour to allow the mixture to firm up.
2 Form the mixture into 12 walnut-sized balls using floured hands, then lightly dust each ball in flour.
3 Heat 1 tablespoon of oil in a non-stick skillet and cook the falafel four at a time (adding more oil when necessary) 6 minutes, turning them occasionally, until golden all over. Drain on paper towels.

tofu bites

Cubes of marinated and roasted golden tofu make great nibbles, an addition to a salad such as the Chinese Noodle Salad (see page 85), or as a filling for wraps and pita breads.

4 tbsp. black bean sauce
1 tbsp. clear honey
1 tbsp. soy sauce
2 tsp. sesame oil

8oz. firm tofu, patted dry and
  cut into ¾in. cubes
sunflower oil, for brushing

1 Mix together the black bean sauce, honey, soy sauce, and sesame oil in a shallow dish. Add the tofu and spoon the marinade over until the tofu is completely covered. Leave to marinate 1 hour, turning the tofu occasionally.
2 Heat the oven to 350°F. Lightly brush a roasting pan with oil. Arrange the tofu in the tin and roast 20 minutes, turning halfway, until golden and slightly crisp all over.

SERVES 4

PREPARATION + COOKING
10 + 20 minutes + marinating

STORAGE
Make in advance and refrigerate for up to 3 days.

SERVE THIS WITH...
Chinese Noodle Salad
  (see page 85)
Summer Pudding (see page 130)
fruit

HEALTH BENEFITS
Tofu is made from the soybean, which is super-nutritious and known as the "meat of the earth" in China, because it is among only a few plant foods that are complete proteins.

*chicken burgers

HEALTH BENEFITS
Chicken is a low-fat source of protein as long as the fatty skin is removed. It is also a good source of the amino acid tryptophan, which is vital for the production of the feel-good brain chemical serotonin.

Low-fat and high in protein, these burgers are delicious cold and can be served either in a bun with relish and the usual accompaniments or solo with a dip such as Tzatziki (see page 34) or Tomato Salsa (see page 30). Instead of chicken, you could use turkey, lean beef, or vegetarian meat crumbles.

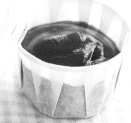

1 small onion
2 tbsp. chopped alfalfa sprouts
1 small carrot, finely grated
1 apple, cored, then grated,
    skin and all
1lb. ground chicken

1 small free-range egg,
    lightly beaten
all-purpose flour, for dusting
salt
freshly ground black pepper
olive oil, for brushing

1 Put the onion, alfalfa sprouts, carrot, apple, and ground chicken in a mixing bowl. Stir or use your hands to break it up and mix everything together.

2 Add the egg and seasoning and mix again by hand.

3 Lightly cover a plate and your hands with flour. Divide the mixture into six and shape each portion into a circular, flat burger. Place the burgers on a plate, cover with plastic wrap and chill 30 minutes.

4 Heat the broiler to medium and line a baking sheet with foil. Lightly brush the foil with oil and place the burgers on top. Brush the top of the burgers with oil and broil about 8 minutes on each side until golden.

MAKES 6

PREPARATION + COOKING
20 + 16 minutes + chilling

STORAGE
Make in advance and refrigerate for up to 3 days or freeze for up to 1 month (unless the chicken was frozen). Keep chilled until ready to eat (see page 11).

SERVE THIS WITH...
seeded burger bun
relish
tomato ketchup
lettuce and sliced tomato
Banana & Blueberry Muffin
  (see page 132)
fruit

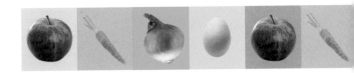

MAKES 6

PREPARATION + COOKING
10 + 12 minutes + chilling

STORAGE
Make in advance and refrigerate for up to 3 days or freeze for up to 1 month. Keep chilled until ready to eat (see page 11).

SERVE THIS WITH...
a bun (with favorite burger accompaniments) or on its own
Italian Flag Salad (see page 80)
Date & Pecan Brownie (see page 133)
fruit

HEALTH BENEFITS
Wholewheat bread is an unrefined carbohydrate food that contains plenty of fiber and will keep your child feeling fuller for longer than white bread would.

tuna patties

Canned tuna makes a convenient lunchbox staple, but instead of the usual sandwich filling here it is an ideal base for a pattie-cum-burger.

2 slices day-old wholewheat bread
7oz. canned lightmeat tuna in spring water, drained well
1 small onion, grated
1 tsp. dried oregano
1 tbsp. all-purpose flour, plus extra for dusting
1 medium free-range egg, beaten
salt
freshly ground black pepper
2 tbsp. sunflower oil

1 Place the bread in a food processor or blender and process into breadcrumbs. Transfer to a mixing bowl with the tuna, onion, oregano, flour, and egg. Season and chill 1 hour to allow the mixture to firm up.

2 Lightly cover a plate and your hands in flour. Divide the tuna mixture into six and form into pattie shapes, then dust with more flour—the mixture is quite loose but will firm up when cooked.

3 Heat half the oil in a skillet and cook three of the patties about 3 minutes on each side until golden, then drain on paper towels. Repeat with the remaining patties, adding more oil if necessary. Let cool before packing in an airtight container, placing a sheet of waxed paper between each pattie.

zucchini & parmesan fritters

These cheesy fritters taste delicious dipped into the Tomato Salsa on page 30. Lightly steamed chunks of broccoli, or peas, or corn can be used instead of the zucchini, if preferred.

8oz. zucchini,
   coarsely grated
3 tbsp. finely grated
   Parmesan cheese
1 free-range egg, beaten

2 tbsp. white all-purpose flour
2 tbsp. sunflower oil
salt
freshly ground black pepper

1 Squeeze the zucchini in a dish-towel to remove any moisture. Mix the zucchini with the Parmesan, egg, and flour, then season.
2 Heat half the oil in a skillet. Add 2 tablespoons of the zucchini mixture for each fritter to make six in total. Cook in two batches for 2–3 minutes on each side until set and golden. Drain on paper towels and let cool.

MAKES 6

PREPARATION + COOKING
15 + 12 minutes

STORAGE
Make in advance and refrigerate for up to 3 days or freeze for up to 1 month.

SERVE THIS WITH...
Tortilla Dippers with Tomato
   Salsa (see page 30)
carrot and celery sticks
Cinnamon-spiced Apples
   (see page 120)

HEALTH BENEFITS
Summer squash such as zucchini are at their best during the warmer months; small ones have a better flavor than large ones.

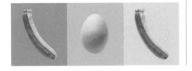

V O

spaghetti frittata

A great way to use up leftover spaghetti, this substantial "omelet" works well in a lunchbox, providing valuable amounts of both protein and carbohydrate.

SERVES 4–6

PREPARATION + COOKING
10 + 20 minutes

STORAGE
Make in advance and refrigerate for up to 3 days.

SERVE THIS WITH...
crusty bread
Mixed Bean Salad (see page 82)
muffin
fruit

HEALTH BENEFITS
Wholewheat or brown pasta is higher in fiber and B vitamins than the white varieties.

3oz. wholewheat or
   white spaghetti
olive oil, for stirring
5 free-range eggs, beaten

2¼oz. Parmesan cheese,
   grated
½oz. butter
salt
freshly ground black pepper

1 Cook the spaghetti in plenty of boiling water, following the package instructions, until al dente. Drain and refresh under cold running water. Tip the pasta into a bowl, stir in a little oil to stop it sticking together, then set aside.

2 Season the beaten eggs and mix in the Parmesan. Heat the broiler to medium.

3 Melt the butter in a medium-size skillet with a heatproof handle. Place the spaghetti in the skillet in an even layer then pour the egg mixture over the pasta. Cook about 5 minutes until the base is set and slightly golden.

4 Place the pan under the broiler and cook the top of the frittata about 3 minutes until set. Let cool, then cut into wedges.

tuna & onion tortilla

Substantial enough to withstand being carried about in a lunchbox, tortillas taste just as good cold as hot. A wedge of tortilla in a crusty roll with some chutney is a fine combination.

1 tbsp. olive oil
1 large onion, sliced
7oz. canned lightmeat tuna, drained

1lb. cooked potatoes, peeled and diced
6 free-range eggs, beaten
salt
freshly ground black pepper

1 Heat the oil in a medium skillet with a heatproof handle, then fry the onion 8 minutes until softened and slightly golden. Stir in the tuna, retaining some chunks, then top with the potatoes, spreading the ingredients evenly.
2 Heat the broiler to medium. Season the eggs and pour them into the skillet. Cook 5 minutes over medium heat until the base is golden and set.
3 Place the skillet under the broiler and cook the tortilla about 3 minutes until set. Cool, then cut into wedges.

SERVES 4–6

PREPARATION + COOKING
10 + 17 minutes

STORAGE
Make in advance and refrigerate for up to 3 days. Keep chilled until ready to eat (see page 11).

SERVE THIS WITH...
Ham, Bean & Pineapple Salad (see page 84)
Carrot Cake (see page 134)
fruit

HEALTH BENEFITS
In natural medicine onions were praised as a "cure-all." Today they are believed to provide potent phytochemicals that may protect against both cancer and heart disease.

vegetable samosas

Light and crisp low-fat phyllo pastry is used to make these lightly spiced Indian pockets.

MAKES 10

PREPARATION + COOKING
25 + 30 minutes

STORAGE
Make in advance and refrigerate for up to 3 days or freeze for up to 1 month.

SERVE THIS WITH...
Carrot, Raisin & Pine Nut Salad (see page 77)
natural yogurt with honey
berries

HEALTH BENEFITS
Little nuggets of goodness, peas are a good source of protein, vitamins B and C, iron, potassium, and phosphorus.

1 tbsp. vegetable oil, plus extra
   for greasing
1 onion, finely chopped
1 carrot, diced
2 large cloves garlic,
   finely chopped
1 tbsp. grated fresh ginger
2 tsp. garam masala
¼ tsp. chili powder (optional)
9oz. cooked new
   potatoes, diced
3 tbsp. frozen petits pois
salt
freshly ground black pepper
6 sheets phyllo pastry

1 Heat the oil in a skillet and fry the onion 3 minutes, then add the carrot and cook another 4 minutes. Add the garlic, ginger, and spices and cook 1 more minute.

2 Stir in the potatoes, peas, and 4 tablespoons of water, cover, and simmer 5 minutes to absorb the water. Season. Place in a bowl to cool. Heat the oven to 375°F.

3 Lightly grease two baking sheets. Take three sheets of phyllo pastry and place them on top of one another. Cut five 6-inch circles and place on a baking sheet. Repeat.

4 Place a heaped tablespoon of filling in the center of one circle, wet the edge of the pastry, and fold it over to make a half-moon shape, sealing the edges well. Brush with oil.

5 Repeat with the remaining circles of phyllo and filling to make 10 samosas. Bake 15 minutes until golden.

spring rolls

Filled with crisp and crunchy vegetables, these spring rolls are baked to keep down fat levels.

2oz. rice vermicelli noodles
2 tsp. sunflower oil, plus extra
   for brushing
1 tsp. toasted sesame oil
2 carrots, cut into thin strips
1 red bell pepper, seeded and
   cut into thin strips
3oz. snow peas, sliced
   diagonally
2 cloves garlic, chopped

2 scallions, finely
   sliced lengthwise
1in. piece fresh ginger, peeled
   and grated
2 tsp. soy sauce
3oz. beansprouts
16 small spring roll wrappers,
   4½in. square, defrosted if
   frozen
1 free-range egg white, beaten

1 Soak the noodles as instructed on the package, drain, and refresh under cold water. Cut into short lengths.
2 Heat the oils in a wok and stir-fry the vegetables 2 minutes. Add the soy sauce and cook another minute. Add the beansprouts. Place in a bowl, stir, and let cool.
3 Heat the oven to 350°F. Put one wrapper at a time on a work surface (covering the rest with a damp dish towel). Place a heaped tablespoon of filling on one corner, fold the corner over it, fold in the two sides and roll the wrapper. Brush the edge with egg white and fold to seal.
4 Place the spring rolls on a lightly oiled baking sheet. Brush each roll with oil and bake 15 minutes until golden.

MAKES 16

PREPARATION + COOKING
25 + 15 minutes

STORAGE
Make in advance and refrigerate for up to 3 days or freeze for up to 1 month.

SERVE THIS WITH...
small cup of plum, soy, or
   sweet chili dipping sauce
Oriental Rice Salad (see page 91)
Apricot & Cashew Nut Bar
   (see page 128)
fruit

HEALTH BENEFITS
These spring rolls are an excellent way to encourage your child to eat a variety of vegetables. Try to provide a variety of colored fresh vegetables, since each color contains a range of healthy phytochemicals or plant nutrients.

*sushi cones

HEALTH BENEFITS
Sea vegetables such as nori are rich in minerals that benefit the nervous system, boost immunity, and help the metabolism.

This may sound a bit complicated or indeed sophisticated for a child's lunchbox, but hand-rolled cones are surprisingly easy and don't need any specialist equipment. They're also fun to make and great for kids to get involved with. Instead of the hot-smoked trout or salmon, try slices of smoked trout, crabsticks, avocado, sweet bell pepper, or cooked chicken.

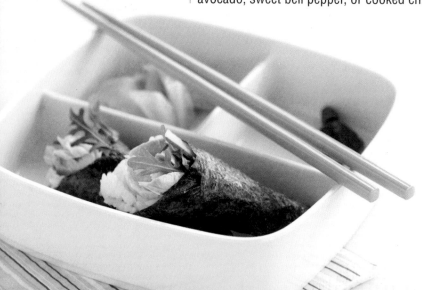

½ cup sushi rice
1½ tbsp. rice vinegar
½ tsp. superfine sugar
¼ tsp. salt
3 sheets nori
2 tbsp. mayonnaise
4 pea-sized amounts wasabi

2¾oz. hot-smoked trout or
   salmon, in large flakes
handful arugula leaves
6 thin sticks cucumber, seeded,
   2in. long
tamari (wheat-free soy sauce)
   and pickled ginger, to serve
   (optional)

MAKES 6

PREPARATION + COOKING
25 + 15 minutes

STORAGE
Make the day before and
refrigerate overnight.

SERVE THIS WITH...
slices of bell pepper
   and celery
Date & Pecan Brownie
   (see page 133)
fruit

1 Put the rice and ¾ cup water in a saucepan.
Bring to a boil, reduce to a simmer, cover, and cook
12–15 minutes until the water is absorbed. Leave
5 minutes, covered.

2 Meanwhile, mix together the rice vinegar, sugar, and salt.
Transfer the rice to a bowl to cool, then gently stir in the
rice vinegar mixture using a wooden spoon. Let cool.

3 Cut the nori sheets into six 4-inch squares. Mix the
mayonnaise and wasabi and smear over each square.

4 Place 2 teaspoons of rice diagonally down the center
of each square. On top lay a few flakes of trout, a few
arugula leaves, and a stick of cucumber. Wet one edge of
the nori and roll into a cone shape; press the edge to seal.

5 Serve with tamari and pickled ginger, if liked.

Hot-smoked
fish has a more
delicate smoky
flavor than cold-
smoked fish and a
firmer texture.

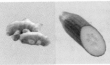

MAKES 8

PREPARATION + COOKING
10 + 20 minutes

STORAGE
Make in advance and refrigerate for up to 3 days or freeze for up to 1 month (unless the turkey was frozen). Keep chilled until ready to eat (see page 11).

SERVE THIS WITH...
Tortilla Dippers with Tomato Salsa (see page 30)
vegetable sticks
Winter Fruit Salad (see page 122)

HEALTH BENEFITS
An excellent low-fat source of protein, turkey also provides immune-boosting zinc as well as selenium.

festive turkey balls

These are very quick and simple to make and make use of a stuffing mix. The balls make an excellent filling for pita bread or a tortilla wrap or can be served on their own dipped into the Tomato Salsa on page 30 or redcurrant sauce.

2½oz. good-quality organic stuffing mix
¾oz. unsalted butter

7oz. turkey breast, diced
olive oil, for brushing

1 Heat the oven to 400°F. Make up the stuffing mix with ⅔ cup just-boiled water and butter following the package instructions. Put the turkey in a food processor and process until very finely chopped. Add the stuffing mix and blend until combined.

2 Roll the mixture into eight balls slightly larger than a walnut and place on an oiled baking sheet. Brush the balls with oil, then bake in the oven about 20 minutes, turning occasionally, until golden and cooked through.

tandoori chicken drumsticks

Children love these lightly spiced chicken drumsticks, which can be eaten with their hands.

2 skinless chicken drumsticks
1 tbsp. lemon juice
5 tbsp. thick natural bio yogurt

2 tbsp. tandoori spice blend
sunflower oil, for brushing

1 Pat the chicken dry with paper towels. Make three deep cuts in each drumstick and rub the lemon juice over them.
2 Put the yogurt and tandoori spices in a shallow dish and mix together. Add the chicken and completely cover with the marinade. Cover and chill at least 1 hour.
3 Heat the oven to 400°F. Brush a baking sheet with oil and add the chicken. Cook in the oven 15 minutes, then turn the chicken over, and spoon over some more of the marinade. Cook another 15 minutes until cooked through with no trace of pinkness inside.

SERVES 2

PREPARATION + COOKING
15 + 30 minutes + marinating

STORAGE
Make the day before and refrigerate. Keep chilled until ready to eat (see page 11).

SERVE THIS WITH...
Spicy Sweet Potatoes
  (see page 95)
sliced cucumber
mango chutney
Banana & Blueberry Muffin
  (see page 132)
fruit

HEALTH BENEFITS
Spices add plenty of flavor to food, but also benefit health in that they help aid digestion and have valuable antibacterial properties.

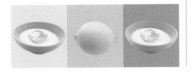

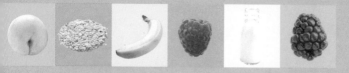

SWEET TREATS & BAKES

These desserts, cakes, and breads have been created with health in mind—with a few concessions to the occasional indulgence. You'll find fresh and dried fruit in various guises, from fruit salads to muffins and cakes, and different takes on the cereal bar, including dates, apricots, and cashews. Some of the sweet treats are sufficiently quick and simple to make on the day, while others need a bit more preparation but will keep for a few days. The Seeded Dough Balls, Cheese Scones, and Oat Crackers make a great alternative to bread while being just as versatile, and are perfect filled or topped with various sweet or savory foods.

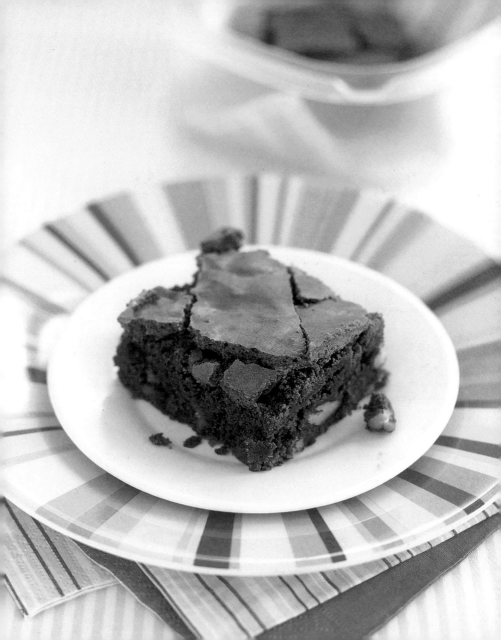

cinnamon-spiced apples

This lightly spiced apple compote can be served on its own, stirred into vanilla custard, or pureed and combined with thick natural yogurt. It freezes well, so can be prepared in bulk and frozen in single portions for later use.

SERVES 2–4

PREPARATION + COOKING
10 + 15 minutes

STORAGE
Make in advance and refrigerate for up to 5 days or freeze for up to 1 month.

SERVE THIS WITH...
Vegetable Samosas
 (see page 112)
Smashed Bean & Carrot Spread
 (see page 33)
vegetable sticks

HEALTH BENEFITS
In natural medicine, apples are renowned for their cleansing properties, and for their ability to aid digestion and remove impurities from the liver.

5 apples, cored, peeled, and
 roughly chopped
1 tsp. ground cinnamon

1 tsp. fresh lemon juice
small knob of butter (optional)

1 Put the apples, cinnamon, lemon juice (this prevents the apples turning brown), butter, if using, and $^2/_3$ cup water in a saucepan. Bring to a boil, then simmer over medium-low heat 12–15 minutes, until the apples are tender.
2 Lightly mash the apples with a fork to break them down slightly, then let cool.

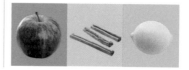

summer fruit salad

The beauty of a fruit salad is that it is infinitely flexible, allowing you to choose favorite fruits and the best of those in season. Try to use a variety of fruit, of different shapes and colors, so that it will not only look good but also contain a range of nutrients.

8 strawberries, hulled and halved or quartered, if large
1 nectarine, pitted and cut into bite-size chunks
1 kiwi fruit, peeled, quartered, and cut into bite-size chunks

1 apple, cored and cut into bite-size chunks
8 seedless grapes, halved
4 tbsp. orange juice

1 Divide the fruit between two lidded containers.
2 Pour 2 tablespoons of orange juice over each fruit salad and cover.

SERVES 2

PREPARATION
10 minutes

STORAGE
Make on the day itself for maximum nutrients, or make the day before and refrigerate.

SERVE THIS WITH...
Honey-sesame Sausages (see page 23)
Creamy Guacamole (see page 31)
pita bread
vegetable sticks

HEALTH BENEFITS
Vitamin levels begin to deplete when fruit is cut, so it's best, if possible, to prepare fruit salad as close to serving as possible for maximum nutrient levels.

winter fruit salad

With flavors reminiscent of Christmas, the cinnamon and cloves add a comforting warmth to this mineral-rich dried fruit salad. If your child finds chunks off-putting, the fruit salad can be pureed with no ill effect to the taste and mixed with natural yogurt.

SERVES 4

PREPARATION + COOKING
10 + 15 minutes

STORAGE
Make in advance and refrigerate for up to 1 week.

SERVE THIS WITH...
Festive Turkey Balls
  (see page 116)
wholewheat tortilla wrap
chutney
Cheesy Celery Stalks
  (see page 22)
cookie

HEALTH BENEFITS
Since dried fruit has a rich concentration of beta-carotene, B vitamins, iron, and potassium and is naturally sweet, no extra sugar is needed.

7oz. mixed dried fruit such as apples, apricots, peaches, prunes, and so on, cut into bite-size pieces

1¼ cups fresh orange juice
1 cinnamon stick
1 star anise
2 cloves

1 Put the dried fruit, orange juice, 6 tablespoons of water, cinnamon, star anise, and cloves in a saucepan. Bring to a boil then reduce the heat, cover, and simmer 10 minutes until the fruit has softened.

2 Remove from the heat, let cool, and divide among four small lidded containers.

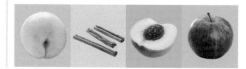

mango fool

For the best-flavored fool, make sure the mango is perfectly ripe and juicy. This creamy dessert is also delicious made with berries, plums or nectarines.

1 mango
scant ½ cup thick natural bio
   yogurt

²/₃ cup low-fat fromage frais
1 tbsp. honey, or to taste
1 tsp. vanilla extract (optional)

1 Peel the mango using a vegetable peeler and slice the fruit off the large central pit. Put the mango in a blender with the rest of the ingredients and blend until smooth and creamy.
2 Transfer the mango fool to two lidded containers.

SERVES 2

PREPARATION
10 minutes

STORAGE
Make in advance and refrigerate for up to 3 days.

SERVE THIS WITH...
Chicken Tikka Naan (see page 66)
cucumber slices and
   cherry tomatoes
cookie for dunking

HEALTH BENEFITS
An excellent source of vitamin C and beta-carotene, mango will benefit hair, skin, and nails.

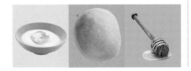

087

*strawberry crunch cup

HEALTH BENEFITS
Energy-giving oats provide useful amounts of fiber and B vitamins. Research shows that foods high in carbohydrates boost the brain's levels of the feel-good chemical serotonin; levels of this tend to fall during the winter.

This is so simple to make and is much healthier than store-bought fruit yogurts—it is also an ideal breakfast or quick dessert. You could quadruple the oat and seed mixture, then store any surplus in an airtight jar for up to a week. If strawberries are out of season, sliced bananas are also good, or you could try frozen berries instead.

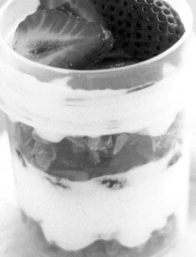

¼ cup quick oats
1 tbsp. sunflower seeds
1 tbsp. pumpkin seeds
1–2 tbsp. clear honey or
    maple syrup

6 heaped tbsp. thick natural
    bio yogurt
½ tsp. vanilla extract
6 strawberries, hulled and
    thickly sliced

SERVES 1

PREPARATION + COOKING
10 + 5 minutes

STORAGE
Make the day before and
refrigerate overnight. The oat
and seed mixture will keep in an
airtight container for 1 week.

SERVE THIS WITH...
Creamy Tomato & Lentil Soup
    (see page 38)
bread
fruit

1 Put the oats in a dry skillet and toast over medium-low
heat 3 minutes, turning the oats occasionally with a
spatula.
2 Next, add the sunflower and pumpkin seeds to the pan
and toast another 2 minutes, tossing the skillet frequently
until the oats and seeds are light golden.
3 Remove the skillet from the heat and stir in the honey or
maple syrup. This will sizzle at first, but keep stirring until
the oats and seeds are coated. Leave to cool slightly to
allow the mixture to crisp up.
4 Mix the yogurt with the vanilla extract.
5 Put a layer of the oat mixture in the bottom of a
tall lidded cup. Top with half the yogurt then half the
strawberries. Repeat with another layer of each. Cover.

Honey is known
for its antiseptic
healing properties.
Since it's sweeter
than sugar, you
need less.

apple flapjacks

Full of energy-giving oats, fruit, and seeds, these granola-type bars are a perfect lunchbox treat.

MAKES 10

PREPARATION + COOKING
15 + 35 minutes

STORAGE
Make in advance and keep in an airtight container for up to 1 week.

SERVE THIS WITH...
Ham & Egg Pie (see page 103)
Carrot, Raisin & Pine Nut Salad
(see page 77)
fruit

HEALTH BENEFITS
Pumpkin seeds are one of the few foods to contain both omega-3 and omega-6 essential fatty acids.

3½oz. unsalted butter, plus
extra for greasing
scant ½ cup light soft brown
sugar
4 tbsp. corn syrup

heaped 2 cups rolled oats
1 tbsp. sesame seeds
1 tbsp. pumpkin seeds
2 tbsp. sunflower seeds
1 apple, cored and grated

1 Heat the oven to 350°F. Grease the sides and line the base of an 8-inch square pan. Melt the butter in a saucepan with the sugar and syrup over low heat, stirring occasionally; do not allow the mixture to boil.

2 Put the oats, seeds, and apple in a mixing bowl and pour in the buttery syrup. Stir until everything is mixed together.

3 Spoon the oat mixture into the prepared pan and bake 25–30 minutes until golden and lightly crisp. Cut into 10 bars while still warm and leave in the pan until cool.

chewy date bars

Cereal bars can be on the dry side, but these have a layer of pureed dates for moistness.

4½oz. unsalted butter, plus
    extra for greasing
1½ cups chopped ready-to-eat
    dried dates
1 cup wholewheat plain flour

1 tsp. baking powder
½ cup light soft brown sugar
generous ½ cup rolled oats
4 tbsp. sunflower seeds

1 Grease the sides and line the base of an 11 x 7-inch baking pan. Put the dates and scant 1 cup of water in a saucepan and bring to a boil. Reduce the heat and simmer, half-covered, 20 minutes until the dates are very soft and the water has been absorbed. Puree the dates in a blender and let cool. Heat the oven to 350°F.
2 Meanwhile, mix together the flour, baking powder, sugar, oats, and seeds in a mixing bowl. Rub in the butter until the mixture is soft and crumbly. Spoon three-quarters into the greased pan and press down to make an even layer.
3 Spoon the date mixture over the oats in an even layer, sprinkle with the remaining oat mixture, and press down lightly. Bake 25 minutes until golden, then leave in the pan to cool. Cut into 16 squares and remove from the pan.

MAKES 16

PREPARATION + COOKING
20 + 45 minutes

STORAGE
Make in advance and keep in an airtight container for up to 1 week.

SERVE THIS WITH...
Spaghetti Frittata (see page 110)
red bell pepper and celery sticks
fruit

HEALTH BENEFITS
The brain needs a constant supply of glucose to function properly. Complex carbohydrates found in the wholewheat flour and oats are the primary source of the brain's energy.

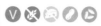

apricot & cashew nut bars

These couldn't be simpler to make and are a wholesome blend of fruit, oats, nuts, and seeds. Replace the nuts with more seeds, if necessary.

MAKES 8

PREPARATION + COOKING
10 + 3 minutes

STORAGE
Make in advance and keep in an airtight container up to 1 week.

SERVE THIS WITH...
Sushi Cones (see page 114)
carrot sticks
fruit yogurt

HEALTH BENEFITS
Rich in B vitamins, vitamin E, iron, calcium, magnesium, and potassium, cashew nuts provide numerous health benefits, but give them to your child in moderation because of their high fat content.

2oz. whole rolled oats
2oz. cashew nuts
5½oz. ready-to-eat dried
    unsulfured apricots, cut into
    small pieces

3½oz. raisins
4 tbsp. fresh orange juice
2 tbsp. sunflower seeds
2 tbsp. pumpkin seeds

1 Put the oats and cashew nuts in a dry skillet and toast them over medium heat 3 minutes, turning occasionally, until they start to turn golden. Let cool.

2 Put the apricots, raisins, and orange juice in a food processor and process to a smooth paste. Scrape the fruit puree into a mixing bowl.

3 Put the oats, nuts and seeds in the food processor and process until finely chopped. Tip the mixture into the bowl with the fruit puree. Stir the fruit mixture until all the ingredients are mixed together.

4 Line a 7 x 10-inch pan with parchment. Tip the mixture into the pan and smooth into an even layer about ½ inch thick. Chill 1 hour, then cut into eight bars.

pancakes with fruit sauce

Pancakes dipped into a smooth strawberry sauce are a great combination and fun to eat.

1¹/₃ cups self-rising flour
2 tsp. superfine sugar
generous ¾ cup milk
1 extra-large free-range egg
vegetable oil, for frying

10½oz. strawberries or mixture of berries
confectioners' sugar, sifted, to taste

Fruit sauce:

1 To make the fruit sauce, process the strawberries in a blender. Press the puree through a strainer to remove any seeds and sweeten with confectioners' sugar to taste.
2 To make the pancakes, sift the flour into a mixing bowl then mix with the sugar. Make a well in the center. Pour the milk into a pitcher, whisk in the egg, then add to the flour and sugar. Beat to make a smooth batter.
3 Heat a little oil in a non-stick skillet and add three small ladlefuls of batter, one for each pancake. Cook about 3 minutes until light golden then turn and cook another 2 minutes. Remove and cook the remaining pancakes.
4 Put the fruit sauce into individual lidded tubs.

MAKES 10 (2 PER PERSON)

PREPARATION + COOKING
10 + 20 minutes

STORAGE
Make in advance and refrigerate for up to 3 days or freeze for up to 1 month.

SERVE THIS WITH...
Corn Chowder (see page 40)
crusty bread
fruit

HEALTH BENEFITS
Strawberries help to boost the immune system thanks to their collection of potent antioxidants. Since the fruit sauce is uncooked, the high levels of vitamin C will remain intact.

HEALTH BENEFITS
Berries are an excellent source of vitamin C, folate, and the antioxidants ellagic acid and quercetin. They are also thought to help prevent cold sores, asthma, and hay fever.

*summer pudding

Packed with juicy summer berries, these little summer puddings don't just look good: they're full of vitamins too. You could use fresh berries, but frozen bags of mixed fruit mean that you can make these fruity desserts at any time of year.

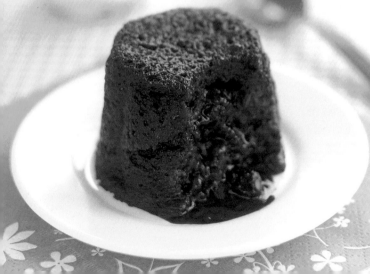

vegetable oil, for greasing
10–12 thin small slices
wholewheat bread,
crusts removed

4 (10-cup) bags frozen summer
berries
6 tbsp. superfine sugar

SERVES 4

PREPARATION + COOKING
15 + 5 minutes

STORAGE
Make in advance and refrigerate
for up to 3 days or freeze for up
to 1 month.

SERVE THIS WITH...
Tuna Quesadilla (see page 65)
cucumber and cherry tomatoes

1 Lightly oil four 5-fluid-ounce dariole molds or small lidded cups. Cut four circles of bread to fit the base of each mold. Cut each of the remaining bread slices into four triangles. Put a bread circle into each mold, then arrange the triangular pieces of bread around the sides, packing them tightly together to avoid any gaps. Allow the bread to overlap the top slightly. Set aside four triangles.

2 Meanwhile, put the fruit in a saucepan with the sugar and ½ cup water and simmer gently 4–5 minutes until the berries are defrosted and very juicy.

3 Spoon a little of the berry juice into each mold, then divide the fruit between the molds, leaving 4 tablespoons of juice to spoon over the puddings.

4 Fold the bread over the fruit filling, then top with the remaining triangles. Spoon over the juice, then cover each pudding with a plate and a weight and refrigerate overnight.

Among their many
health benefits,
berries are a good
source of lutein,
which is important
for healthy vision.

banana & blueberry muffins

These muffins will give pre-lunch depleted blood-sugar levels a welcome boost.

MAKES 10

PREPARATION + COOKING
15 + 20 minutes

STORAGE
Make the day before and keep in an airtight container. Muffins are best eaten as fresh as possible.

SERVE THIS WITH...
Chicken Strips with Satay Dip (see page 26)
pita bread
carrot sticks and cherry tomatoes
fruit

HEALTH BENEFITS
A superfood, blueberries are rich in powerful antioxidants called anthocyanins, which mop up potentially harmful free radicals in the body.

2 cups white all-purpose flour
pinch of salt
1 tsp. baking powder
²/₃ cup superfine sugar
¹/₃ cup milk

2 free-range eggs
5oz. unsalted butter, melted
2 bananas, mashed
1 cup blueberries

1 Heat the oven to 400°F. Place 10 large paper baking cups in a deep muffin pan.
2 Sift the flour, salt, and baking powder into a bowl, stir in the sugar, and mix together. Make a well in the center.
3 Put the milk, eggs, and butter in a pitcher and whisk until combined. Add to the bowl with the bananas, stir just to combine, then fold in the blueberries. Spoon into the pan.
4 Bake 20 minutes until risen. Cool on a wire rack.

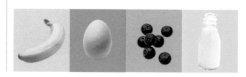

date & pecan brownies

These fruit-and-nut chocolate brownies make a perfect treat. Leave the pecans out if necessary.

heaped ½ cup pecans, broken
   in half
5½oz. dark chocolate, broken
   into chunks
5½oz. unsalted butter,
   cut into pieces
scant 1½ cups
   superfine sugar

3 free-range eggs,
   lightly beaten
1 cup white all-purpose flour
1½ tsp. baking powder
3½oz. dried ready-to-eat dates,
   cut into small pieces

1 Heat the oven to 350°F. Line and grease an 8-inch square cake pan. Put the pecans on a baking sheet and roast about 5 minutes until they are slightly golden and smell toasted.

2 Meanwhile, melt the chocolate and butter in a bowl over a pan of slightly simmering water, stirring very occasionally. Remove from the heat and let cool slightly.

3 Whisk together the sugar and eggs in a bowl until pale and stir into the chocolate mixture. Sift in the flour and baking powder, then add the pecans and dates. Mix with a wooden spoon, then pour into the prepared pan.

4 Cook 40–45 minutes until the top forms a light crust, but the center is still slightly gooey. Let cool in the pan then turn out and cut into 12 squares.

MAKES 12

PREPARATION + COOKING
15 + 50 minutes

STORAGE
Make in advance and keep in an airtight container for up to 1 week.

SERVE THIS WITH...
Cheese, Apple & Chutney Bun
  (see page 52)
carrot and bell pepper sticks
fruit

HEALTH BENEFITS
Dates are a rich source of fiber and are high in potassium and contain some iron, while pecans contain protein, iron, calcium, and fiber.

MAKES 15 SQUARES

PREPARATION + COOKING
20 + 50 minutes

STORAGE
Make in advance and keep in an airtight container for up to 1 week.

SERVE THIS WITH…
Corn Chowder (see page 40)
wholewheat pita bread
fruit

HEALTH BENEFITS
Recent research has found that, along with bountiful amounts of beneficial nutrients, carrots may help to protect against food poisoning.

carrot cake

This is one of the easiest cakes in the world to make, but it's still incredibly light and moist.

butter, for greasing
heaped 1 cup wholewheat self-rising flour
heaped 1 cup white self-rising flour
2 tsp. ground mixed spice
heaped 1 cup light soft brown sugar

9oz. carrots, grated
4 free-range eggs, lightly beaten
generous ¾ cup sunflower oil

Icing:
½ cup low-fat cream cheese
5 tbsp. confectioners' sugar
1 tsp. vanilla extract

1 Heat the oven to 350°F. Grease the sides and line the base of an 8-inch square cake pan.
2 Sift the flours into a mixing bowl, adding the bran left in the sifter. Stir in the spice, sugar, and carrots and combine thoroughly.
3 Add the eggs and oil, then stir until all the ingredients are combined. Pour into the pan and smooth the top. Bake 50 minutes until risen and golden. Leave in the pan 10 minutes, then turn out on to a rack and let cool.
4 Beat the cream cheese and confectioners' sugar in a mixing bowl until smooth and creamy. Stir in the vanilla extract. Chill 10 minutes then spread over the cake and smooth with a palette knife. Cut into 15 squares.

custard tartlets

These mini custard tarts make a great treat in a lunchbox. What's more, the pastry is phyllo, which is lower in fat than shortcrust or puff and needs no preparation.

3 sheets phyllo pastry,
  defrosted if frozen
¾oz. butter, melted
2 extra-large free-range eggs

3 tbsp. superfine sugar
1¼ cups milk
1 tsp. vanilla extract
freshly grated nutmeg

MAKES 8

PREPARATION + COOKING
10 + 20 minutes

STORAGE
Make in advance and refrigerate for up to 3 days.

SERVE THIS WITH...
Pesto Pasta Salad (see page 86) fruit

HEALTH BENEFITS
Eggs are packed with nutrients, including protein, vitamins A, D, E, and the B group, as well as the minerals iron, phosphorus, and zinc.

1 Heat the oven to 375°F. Place the sheets of phyllo on top of one another and cut into eight 4½-inch squares.
2 Lightly brush eight cups of a deep muffin pan with melted butter, then place a three-layered square of filo pastry in each one. Press the phyllo into each cup, leaving the top to overhang the tin. Brush the top of the phyllo with the rest of the melted butter.
3 Beat together the eggs and sugar in a bowl. Heat the milk, then pour it into the egg mixture with the vanilla and beat again. Strain the mixture into a pitcher then pour into the pastry shells. Grate a little nutmeg over the top.
4 Bake the tartlets about 20 minutes until the pastry is golden and the filling set. Transfer to a wire rack to cool.

apricot cookies

These tempting cookies contain nutritious oats and apricots.

2½oz. light soft brown sugar
4½oz. unsalted butter, softened and cubed
½ cup white self-rising flour
¼ cup wholewheat self-rising flour
½ cup rolled oats
5 ready-to-eat dried apricots, cut into small pieces

1 Heat the oven to 350°F. Line two baking sheets with baking paper.
2 Cream the sugar and butter together in a mixing bowl until light and fluffy. Fold in both types of flour, the oats, and apricots and beat until creamy.
3 Divide the mixture into 10 pieces and roll each one into a ball. Arrange on the prepared baking sheets, well spaced out to allow for the cookies to spread. Flatten the top of each ball slightly and bake 15–20 minutes until just golden but still slightly soft in the centers.
4 Transfer the cookies to a wire rack to cool.

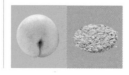

oat crackers

These crackers are very popular served on their own, spread with jam or cream cheese, or with a chunk of cheese, or a slice of ham.

vegetable oil, for greasing
1 cup pinhead oats
²/₃ cup wholewheat plain flour,
    plus extra for dusting
1 tsp. baking powder

pinch of salt
1¾oz. butter, diced
1 tbsp. superfine sugar
2 tbsp. milk

1 Heat the oven to 400°F. Lightly grease a baking sheet.
2 Sift the oats, flour, and baking powder into a mixing bowl, adding any bran left in the sieve. Add the salt and stir until combined.
3 Rub the butter and sugar into the flour mixture using fingertips until it resembles breadcrumbs. Pour in the milk and mix with a fork and then your hands to make a dough.
4 Turn the dough on to a lightly floured work surface and knead briefly until smooth. Using a floured rolling pin, roll out the dough into a rectangle about ¼ inch thick. Trim the edges and cut into 12 squares, re-rolling as necessary.
5 Place the oat biscuits on the baking sheet and prick the tops of the biscuits with a fork. Bake 10 minutes until light golden. Transfer to a wire rack to cool.

MAKES 12

PREPARATION + COOKING
15 + 10 minutes

STORAGE
Make in advance and keep in an airtight container up to 1 week.

SERVE THIS WITH...
chunk of cheese or slice of ham
Creamy Tomato & Lentil Soup
  (see page 38)
fruit yogurt
fruit

HEALTH BENEFITS
Oats are a low-GI complex carbohydrate, meaning that they are absorbed slowly into the bloodstream and have a stabilizing effect on blood-sugar levels, thus insuring sustained amounts of energy.

V O

cheese scones

Savory scones make a tasty alternative to sandwiches in a lunchbox. These cheesy ones are good on their own or with soup or a salad. Alternatively, fill with crispy bacon, ham, cream cheese and chives, or a filling of your choice.

MAKES 10

PREPARATION
10 + 12 minutes

STORAGE
Make in advance and keep in an airtight container for up to 3 days or freeze for up to 1 month.

SERVE THIS WITH...
Creamy Tomato & Lentil Soup (see page 38)
Apricot & Cashew Nut Bar (see page 128)
fruit

HEALTH BENEFITS
Extra-virgin olive oil is used instead of butter to make these scones, providing beneficial monounsaturated fat rather than saturated fat. Monounsaturated fat does not lower blood cholesterol but is good at maintaining levels of "good" cholesterol in the body.

1¼ cups white self-rising flour
9 tbsp. wholewheat self-rising flour
½ tsp. baking powder
3½oz. mature cheddar cheese, grated

2 tbsp. extra-virgin olive oil
6–7 tbsp. milk, plus extra for brushing
1 extra-large free-range egg, beaten

1 Heat the oven to 425°F. Lightly dust a baking sheet with flour. Sift both types of flour and baking powder into a mixing bowl, adding any bran left in the sieve. Stir in the cheddar and make a well in the center.

2 Pour in the oil, milk, and egg and mix with a palette knife to form a soft dough. Add a little extra milk if the dough seems dry. Transfer the dough to a lightly floured work surface and knead briefly until smooth.

3 Roll out the dough into a rectangle about 1 inch thick then cut into 10. Arrange the scones on the baking sheet and brush the tops with a little milk. Bake 10–12 minutes until risen and golden.

seeded dough balls

Dunk these into soup, hummus, guacamole, or a bean dip or serve with a salad.

generous 1¹/₃ cups tepid water
2 tsp. dried yeast
3 cups strong white bread flour
1¼ cups strong wholewheat
   bread flour
1½ tsp. salt
5 tbsp. toasted sunflower seeds
olive oil, for brushing

MAKES 20

PREPARATION + COOKING
25 + 20 minutes + rising

STORAGE
Make in advance and keep in an airtight container for up to 5 days or freeze for up to 1 month.

SERVE THIS WITH...
Italian Flag Salad (see page 80)
carrot sticks
Summer Fruit Salad
  (see page 121)

HEALTH BENEFITS
Omega-6 essential fatty acids, calcium, zinc, magnesium, and vitamin E are found in beneficial amounts in sunflower seeds.

1 Pour 6 tablespoons of water into a small bowl. Sprinkle in the yeast, stir until dissolved, and set aside 5 minutes. Sift the flours and salt into a large bowl. Stir in the seeds.
2 Make a well in the center of the flour and pour in the yeast mixture and 1 cup water. Gradually stir in the flour from the sides of the well. Stir in 3–4 tablespoons of water, if necessary, to make a soft dough.
3 Turn the dough out on to a lightly floured work surface. Knead 10 minutes until smooth and elastic. Put in a new bowl and cover with a dish towel. Leave 1½–2 hours.
4 Heat the oven to 425°F. Press the dough with your knuckles, then divide into 20 pieces. Flatten each piece slightly, fold it over, then roll into a ball in your palm. Place on a floured baking sheet and leave 10 minutes.
5 Brush with olive oil and bake 15–20 minutes until risen and golden. Cool on a wire rack.

menu plans

wheat- & gluten-free 5-day menu

A wheat- and gluten-free diet was once thought to be restrictive and nutrient deficient, but we now have a greater understanding of special dietary needs, and food manucturers are offering far more choice than before. Some sauces and condiments are unsuitable, so check labels.

Day 1
Tuna & Onion Tortilla (see page 111)
wheat-/gluten-free wholewheat bread
red bell pepper and cucumber sticks
Summer Fruit Salad (see page 121)

Day 2
Rice Paper Rolls (see page 73)
Super Salad (see page 81)
Mango Fool (see page 123)
fruit

Day 3
Smoked Mackerel, Apple & Potato Salad
    (see page 96)
wheat-/gluten-free crackers

chunk of cheese
natural yogurt and honey
fruit

Day 4
Melon & Halloumi Salad (see page 78)
wheat-/gluten-free flatbread
vegetable sticks, such as carrot, bell
    pepper, cucumber, or celery
Winter Fruit Salad (see page 122)

Day 5
Spicy Carrot & Lentil Soup (see page 41)
Pear & Ham Bundles (see page 24)
wheat-/gluten-free wholewheat roll
fruit

vegetarian 5-day menu

This menu follows the basic principles of a vegetarian diet: to avoid meat, poultry, and fish and any food that contains ingredients derived from an animal, such as gelatin in jelly or animal rennet in some cheeses.

Day 1
Creamy Tomato & Lentil Soup (see page 38)
Seeded Dough Balls (see page 139) or bread
chunk of vegetarian cheese
Banana & Blueberry Muffin (see page 132)
grapes

Day 2
Vegetable Samosa (see page 112)
Carrot, Raisin & Pine Nut Salad (see page 77)
Cinnamon-spiced Apples (see page 120)
milk

Day 3
Spaghetti Frittata (see page 110)
Tortilla Dippers with Tomato Salsa
   (see page 30)
green salad
Apricot Cookies (see page 136)
fruit

Day 4
BBQ Tofu Baguette (see page 54)
Creamy Guacamole (see page 31)
vegetable sticks
natural yogurt with honey
fruit

Day 5
Falafel & Hummus Lavash (see page 68)
Tabbouleh (see page 90)
carrot sticks
fruit
chocolate milk

vegan 5-day menu

This menu follows the basic principles of a vegan diet: to avoid any animal-derived food, such as meat, poultry, and seafood, as well as ingredients that are a by-product of animals, including dairy produce and honey. This does not mean that a vegan diet is restrictive, but you need to insure that your child is getting a healthy mix of vital nutrients.

Day 1
Soy-coated Nuts & Seeds (see page 20)
Miso & Tofu Broth (see page 43), using
    rice noodles
Apricot & Cashew Nut Bar (see page 128)
fruit

Day 2
BBQ Tofu Baguette (see page 54), using
    maple syrup/sweet chili sauce instead
    of honey
cherry tomatoes
Winter Fruit Salad (see page 122)

Day 3
Roasted Red Bell Pepper Hummus
    (see page 28)
breadsticks
selection of vegetable sticks

Savory Spicy Popcorn (see page 21)
soy yogurt
fruit

Day 4
Spicy Bulgur Salad with Nectarines
    (see page 92)
Smashed Bean & Carrot Spread
    (see page 33)
pita bread
fruit

Day 5
Vegetable Samosa (see page 112)
Spicy Sweet Potatoes (see page 95),
    using soy yogurt
Apple Flapjack (see page 126), using
    vegetable margarine instead of butter
fruit

nut-free 5-day menu

A large number of people suffer from some form of allergy, and an allergy to nuts is becoming increasingly common. As the symptoms of this allergy are usually life-threatening, it's vital that nut-allergy sufferers avoid any contact with nuts and by-products, which is why many schools now have a ban on nuts and related foods. Always check food labels.

Day 1
Smashed Bean & Carrot Spread
   (see page 33)
chunk of cheese
Oat Cracker (see page 137)
cherry tomatoes
Summer Fuit Salad (see page 121)

Day 2
Chicken Noodle Soup (see page 46)
wholewheat bread
Custard Tartlet (see page 135)
fruit

Day 3
Sardines & Tomato on Brown (see page 57)
Apple Coleslaw (see page 76)
natural yogurt with honey
fruit

Day 4
Sausage & Barley Salad (see page 94)
carrot sticks
hard-boiled egg
fruit

Day 5
Calzone (see page 101)
green salad
Banana & Blueberry Muffin (see page 132)
fruit

INDEX